Drugs and Social Context

Telmo Mota Ronzani
Editor

Drugs and Social Context

Social Perspectives on the Use of Alcohol and Other Drugs

Springer

Editor
Telmo Mota Ronzani
Department of Psychology
Universidade Federal de Juiz de Fora
Juiz de Fora, Minas Gerais, Brazil

ISBN 978-3-319-72445-4 ISBN 978-3-319-72446-1 (eBook)
https://doi.org/10.1007/978-3-319-72446-1

Library of Congress Control Number: 2018930098

Printed on acid-free paper

This Springer imprint is published by Springer Nature
The registered company is Springer International Publishing AG
The registered company address is: Gewerbestrasse 11, 6330 Cham, Switzerland

I dedicate this book to my loved ones,
Fabiana, Vítor, and Cecilia.

To my children:

Ser sombra (do) presente,
Norte do futuro,
Um quadro velho na parede.
A-presento-me, discretamente,
Olhos no futuro das montanhas de sua vida.

O que ensinar e o que aprender?.
Que não estamos e somos sozinhos?.
De indignar-se com a injustiça?.
E celebrar a vida como eternas crianças?.
Aprendendo, sempre?.
Talvez a resposta seja:
Sou apenas um velho e marcado espelho,
Uma imagem manchada daquilo que estar
por vir,
De forma mais bela, em eterna imperfeição.

Foreword

An opinion on the book *Drugs and Social Context – Social Perspectives on the Use of Alcohol and Other Drugs,*" organized by Telmo Mota Ronzani, is not an easy task.

It is not easy to talk about a book with this title, where "drug" is not even defined. Within, there is no classification of drugs, their receptors are not addressed (pre- and postsynaptic, inhibitors, etc.), and no attention has been given to the biochemical complexities of synthesis or the release of agonist receptors. Also unmentioned are details of these agonists, the wide clinical use of both natural and synthetic agonists, and the drug antagonists of these agonists.

Thus, the book by Ronzani and colleagues is a striking contrast to an "official truth." It emphasizes knowledge of the environment, with its myriad types of knowledge, and factors that constitute the social environment; in fact, it is the path that psychiatry should follow in its studies and conclusions. However, this is not the place to address the great importance of economic sectors that have led psychiatric ideology to other paths.

This book stresses the imperative need to emphasize the impact of the environment on modeling the neurons of the brain, making them a consequence of this fundamental aspect. We almost always ignore the social environment, which should be the main factor that deserves our attention.

I begin discussing this book by saying that its reading reminded me of my time in elementary school, in São José do Rio Preto city, São Paulo state. At that distant time, poetry in Portuguese was a mandatory subject at school, including important discussions in different areas. I remember, in elementary school at 12–14 years old, a poem that the teacher demanded we knew by heart:

Oh! Bendito o que semeia
Livros... livros à mão cheia...
E manda o povo pensar!
O livro caindo n'alma
É germe – que faz a palma
É chuva – que faz o mar.

This book was prepared and written by 19 researchers, associated with departments or services in 14 universities or institutes (in Brazil, USA, Uruguay, and Spain) that study human behavior based on psychiatric characteristics. There are many themes addressed by the authors, some of which are listed below:

Capitalism	Stigmatization
Treatment access	Social withdrawal
Prohibition	Morals
Social stigma	Hygienist ideas
Stereotypes	Harm reduction
Prejudice	Poverty
Discrimination	War on Drugs
Stigma	Oppression
Self-esteem	Alcohol
Moralization	Criminalization
Race	Gender
Vulnerability	Racism

This set of factors, among others, is one of the most fundamental in influencing human behavior, causing it to react in different ways and bringing great psychic suffering that is manifested by a change in thought and behavior.

Therefore, knowing the social environment (often disrespectful and aggressive) better may cause changes that can lead to behavioral modification. It is up to psychiatrists to be aware of this fact, and this book is a good resource for achieving this desideratum.

October, 23rd, 2017 Elisaldo Araújo Carlini
Professor Emeritus
UNIFESP/EPM
São Paulo, SP, Brazil

Preface

Science as Political Action: It Is Just another Book about Drugs

At first glance, the reader may ask, "Why one more book about drugs?" At least that was the question I asked myself when I considered editing this book. The topic "drugs" is already widely discussed in several contexts. We all have more or less well-defined beliefs about the use of psychoactive substances. Regardless of whether we are users, legal or illegal drug sellers, politicians, public managers, or scientists, we use such beliefs to base our actions and positions regarding the topic, whether religious, ideological, or even scientific.

As we look back over the last few centuries, when we defined drugs as a problem and were clearly more focused on their use, it seems that despite some advances and findings, we are still far from having a clear understanding about drugs or a solution to the problem. The complexity of the topic leads to different points of view about the supposed "problem" and its possible solutions, leading to different causal attributions and even adding characteristics to drugs that go beyond their properties. Although we know so many different things about this particular subject, we may not know as much as we think.

Even with recent advances in pharmacology and neurosciences, there is still a *black box* regarding how we develop prevention, treatment, and public policy actions on drugs. The various technical manuals, clinical protocols, and public policies (supposedly supported by scientific data) still seem far from responding to the needs of the drug field. Maybe it is because we still have very limited answers. In general, our focus has been limited to individual aspects, with biological or psychological explanations about substance use. I do not consider these aspects to be the problem. However, it is important to draw attention to the fact no organism or psychological aspect is isolated from the social environment. Therefore, moving away from the antagonism between biological/psychological/sociological viewpoints, it is important to consider the integration between such dimensions. However, this is not the ethereal position of biopsychosocial discourse, which is often general to immobilism, a conceptual inconsistency that gives a false lack of tension in this discussion.

We know from the beliefs and many interests related to drugs that this is an extremely controversial area, with several tensions that have served (and still serve) to legitimize many actions against people and peoples. In this sense, this book assumes the view that individuals are the actors and the result of their own history, which influences and is directly influenced by their social relations. To understand the process of establishing relationships with an individuals' body and subjectivity, it is fundamental to understand their social and cultural relations.

Drugs have different meanings. Through the discourse that drugs are the cause of social problems, the legitimation of criminalization, punishment, and exclusion of a groups' rights are used as a pretext for social cleansing actions and xenophobia in different parts of the world. At this historic moment of a new wave of conservatism in the world, it is important to draw attention to certain discourses that seek to justify penalization and social injustice as if they were neutral discourses, often used with false scientific support. As Karl Marx said, "history repeats itself, the first time as tragedy, the second as farce." That is why it is important to resist and draw attention to the discourses used in this field. It is therefore important to be aware that "science" can and should be a political act for the defense of life and equality among people. Otherwise, we merely repeat socially empty rituals or serve as supporters of the process of oppression and social injustice.

In other words, that is why we are writing another book about drugs. This time, we aim to discuss and deepen knowledge of macro-social relations related to drug use and understand how this area has served as a mechanism of control, exploitation, and maintenance of exclusion. With this goal, we invited authors from different knowledge areas, some not necessarily specialists in the drug field, with the challenge to relate large social issues to drug use. In this perspective, the book was organized in two axes and seven chapters. The first part, "Drugs and Society," presents chapters discussing general aspects of the social basis of substance use. The second part, "Drugs and Social Issues," more specifically looks at social markers such as gender, social class, and race and includes a chapter on territory.

For the opening section, I have written the chapter "The Context of Drug Use in the Consumer Society," which introduces the following topics. I demonstrate how, historically, actions of restriction or incentive regarding the production and consumption of certain drugs are related to commercial gain and the control of certain groups, often justified by the public health discourse. In addition, I criticize the danger of assuming an automatic liberal discourse on drug use and the idea of the citizen-consumer, with a critique of the consumer society model. In the chapter "The Stigmatization of Drug Use as Mechanism of Legitimation of Exclusion," de Silveira, Tostes, Wan, Ronzani, and Corrigan discuss the fact that drug use is one of the most stigmatized behaviors in the world and how this results in a barrier to seeking care and legitimizes exclusion, as well as the punishment of people linked to certain drugs. In "Social Effects of Prohibitionism in the Americas and New Drug Policies," Rossal presents some consequences of actions against drugs based on prohibitionism. The chapter gives examples such as the processes used in Uruguay and some US states for regulating the sale of marijuana.

The section "Drugs and Social Issues" starts with the chapter "Drugs and Poverty: Interfaces of Oppression in the Capitalist World," in which Ximenes, Paiva, Moura Jr., and Costa discuss how the capitalist system generates situations of poverty and how drug consumption is related to processes of oppression, mainly through the criminalization of poverty through the discourse of control of drug use. In "Drugs and Gender," Nuria Romo-Avilés discusses the specificities related to drug use from the gender perspective and draws attention to the idea of appropriate public policies for considering such an aspect. In the chapter "Drugs and Race," Matsumoto, Farias, and Almeida present the concept of racism and how it relates to the strategy of the "war on drugs" and the use of repressive policies in the maintenance of oppression and criminalization of certain populations according to racial markers. Finally, in the chapter "(Des)Occupation of Urban and Rural Spaces, Gentrification, and Drug Use," Dimenstein, Dalla Vecchia, Macedo, and Bastos call attention to the scenes and territories of use as an important element in understanding the consumption of drugs and how this aspect is related to the formulation of public policies.

We do not intend to propose a "solution" to the issue of drugs, because we would have to define better what, in fact, the problem of drug use among people is. As we hope to show in this work, it seems that there are many problems, with various intentions to find solutions or at least to justify actions that seem to have other targets. In summary, we seek to bring out aspects that are not new, but perhaps forgotten or neglected. Thus, perhaps we should talk more about the same topics, so that we do not repeat the farce of history. This is our proposal for another book about drugs, or beyond them...

Juiz de Fora, Minas Gerais, Brazil — Telmo Mota Ronzani

Contents

About the Authors

Silvio Luiz de Almeida, Lawyer. PhD in philosophy and general theory of law from the Faculty of Law of the University of São Paulo. Professor of Law at Mackenzie Presbyterian University, at the undergraduate and postgraduate program in political and economic law. Executive Director of the Luiz Gama Institute. E-mail: silviovlq@gmail.com

Nuria Romo Avilés, Sociologist. PhD in social anthropology. Professor at Department of Social Anthropology at the University of Granada (Spain). Teaches anthropology of health and illness. Coordinator of national and international research projects related to her specialization in studies concerning gender, health, and drug use. Email: nromo@ugr.es

Francisco Inacio Bastos, Graduated in medicine from the State University of Rio de Janeiro (1981). Master's degree in collective health at the State University of Rio de Janeiro (1988) and doctorate in public health at the Oswaldo Cruz Foundation (1995). Postdoctoral/visiting research internships in Germany (1995), Canada (1998), USA (2010), and UK (2003, 2013, 2015). Honorary researcher at Imperial College, London, UK. Scholarship on productivity research on CNPq - level 1A. Develops research on epidemiology and drug use and HIV/AIDS prevention. E-mail: francisco.inacio.bastos@hotmail.com

Patrick W. Corrigan, Distinguished Professor of Psychology at the Illinois Institute of Technology and Principal Investigator of the National Consortium on Stigma and Empowerment (www.NCSE1.org). Editor of *Stigma and Health*, a journal published by the American Psychological Association. E-mail: corrigan@iit.edu

Pedro Henrique Antunes da Costa, Psychologist. PhD in psychology from the Federal University of Juiz de Fora. Researcher at the Center for Research, Intervention and Evaluation for Alcohol and Drugs (CREPEIA). Professor of Psychology at the Machado Sobrinho College. Develops research and practice on topics such as social psychology, community psychology, public health, community health, and public policy. Email: phantunes.costa@gmail.com

Magda Dimenstein, Psychologist. Titular teacher in the Federal University of Rio Grande do Norte (UFRN). Graduated in psychology at UFPE (1986), Master's degree in clinical psychology at PUC/RJ (1994) and doctorate in mental health at the Psychiatric Institute of UFRJ (1998). Postdoctoral internship in Alcalá de Henares University, Spain. Professor of postgraduate psychology program at UFRN. Coordinator of the research group "Subjectivity Modes, Public Policy, and Vulnerability Contexts." Scholarship in productivity research on CNPq - level 1A. President of the board of ANPEPP (2016–2018 administration). E-mail: mgdimenstein@gmail.com.

Marcio Farias, Psychologist. Center for Afro-American Studies (Nepafro)/Afro Brazil Museum. Master's degree and doctorate in progress in social psychology at PUC-SP (2015). Coordinator of the Center for African American Studies (Nepafro). Visiting Professor of the Jesuit Faculty of Philosophy and Theology. Contributor to the Amma Psyche and Negritude Institute. Composes the coordination team of the Education Center of the Afro Brazil Museum. Counselor of the Luiz Gama Institute. Member of Commissions for the Evaluation of Affirmative Actions in Public Tenderings for the Carlos Chagas Foundation. Cultural and Artistic Projects Designer at National Arts Foundation (Funarte). E-mail: t_mfarias@hotmail.com

João Paulo Macedo, Psychologist. Professor of Federal University of Piauí (UFPI). Graduated in psychology from the Santo Agostinho University (2004). Master's degree (2007) and doctorate (2011) in psychology at UFRN. Part of the postgraduate programs in psychology and the Public Policy Postgraduate Program of UFPI, advising master's and doctorate students. Acts in the area of collective health and mental health, with a focus on psychologists' education and practice in public policy and aspects related to the interiorization of the profession and actions in rural contexts. E-mail: mpamacedo@gmail.com

Adriana Eiko Matsumoto, Psychologist. Department of Psychology, Fluminense Federal University. Doctorate in social psychology at the Pontifical Catholic University of São Paulo (PUC/SP). Master's degree in educational psychology at PUC/SP. E-mail: drieiko@yahoo.com.br

James Ferreira Moura Jr, Psychologist. Professor of the University for International Integration of the Afro-Brazilian Lusophony (UNILAB) and of the postgraduate psychology program at the Federal University of Ceará. PhD in psychology from the Federal University of Rio Grande do Sul. Coordinates the Network for Studies and Confrontations of Poverty, Discrimination and Resistance (reaPODERE) of UNILAB. Conducts research on topics such as poverty, discrimination, and shame/humiliation. E-mail: jamesferreirajr@gmail.comunilab.edu.br

Fernando Santana de Paiva, Psychologist. PhD in psychology (social psychology) from the Federal University of Minas Gerais (UFMG). Professor of the Department of Psychology of the Federal University of Juiz de Fora (UFJF). Develops research on topics such as community psychology, political psychology, public policies and human rights, social inequalities, and poverty and drugs. E-mail: fernandosantana.paiva@yahoo.com.br

Telmo Mota Ronzani, Psychologist. Master's degree in social psychology, PhD in health science from the Federal University of São Paulo, and postdoctoral training from the University of Connecticut Health Center. Professor of the Department of Psychology of the Federal University of Juiz de Fora (UFJF). Chair of the Center for Research, Intervention and Evaluation for Alcohol and Drugs (CREPEIA). Scholarship PQ-2 CNPq. E-mail: tm.ronzani@gmail.com

Marcelo Rossal, Anthropologist. Full-time assistant professor and researcher at the Universidad de la República (Uruguay), Department of Social Anthropology and Center for Latin American Interdisciplinary Studies. Bachelor's, master's, and doctoral degrees in social anthropology (Universidad de la República). Currently investigating drug policy, state violence, and treatment for problematic drug use. E-mail: mrossal@fhuce.edu.uy

Pollyanna Santos da Silveira, Psychologist. PhD in health sciences from the Federal University of São Paulo. Professor of Psychology at the Catholic University of Petrópolis. Researcher at the Center for Research, Intervention and Evaluation for Alcohol and Drugs (CREPEIA). Works especially on the stigma of addiction and mental illness. E-mail: pollyannassilveira@gmail.com

Joanna Gonçalves Andrade de Tostes, Psychologist. PhD student at Federal University of Juiz de Fora (UFJF). Researcher at the Center for Research, Intervention and Evaluation for Alcohol & Drugs (CREPEIA). Works especially on the stigma of addiction and mental illness, drug use prevention, treatment and care, social reintegration, and mental health. E-mail: joanna@tostes.org

Marcelo Dalla Vecchia, Psychologist. Master's degree and doctorate in collective health (Unesp/Botucatu). Professor of the Psychology Department of the Federal University of São João Del-Rei (UFSJ). Coordinator of the Drug Policy Research and Intervention Group (NUPID). Part of the postgraduate psychology program at UFSJ, advising the line of research "Institutions, Health, and Society." Part of the editorial commission of the *Gerais: Revista Interinstitucional de Psicologia* magazine. First Secretary of the Brazilian Social Psychology Association (Abrapso) - Regional Minas. E-mail: mdvecchia@ufsj.edu.br

Hoi Ting Wan, Psychologist. Researcher at the University of Illinois. Works especially on stigma and mental health. E-mail: cheryl_281230@yahoo.com.hk

Verônica Morais Ximenes, Psychologist. PhD in psychology from the University of Barcelona (Spain) and postdoctoral degree from the Federal University of Rio Grande do Sul. Associate Professor of undergraduate and graduate programs in psychology at the Federal University of Ceará (UFC). Coordinator of the Nucleus of Community Psychology (NUCOM) of the UFC. Scholarship PQ-2 CNPq. Develops research and practice on topics such as community psychology, psychosocial implications of poverty, public policies, and community development. E-mail: vemorais@yahoo.com.br

Part I
Drugs and Society

Chapter 1
The Context of Drug Use in the Consumer Society

Telmo Mota Ronzani

Abstract This introductory chapter outlines the social bases related to drug use. First, the parallel between capitalist development and the commercial exploitation of drug use is discussed, demonstrating how, historically, such substances were an important source of capital and the reason for exploration of certain territories. Next, it is shown how moral codes have been created that bind certain groups to some substances, consequently legitimizing processes of punishment and oppression against those groups. Moreover, within the modern model of society based on consumption, the logic of the citizen-consumer is described, as well as the processes of separation between those who have access to this benefit and those that do not. This also creates a differentiation between drugs whose use is encouraged and drugs related to certain groups and, therefore, prohibited by the State. Finally, attention is drawn to the importance of understanding macrosocial factors and social determinants related to drug use.

1.1 Introduction

It is well known that psychoactive substances have been used by humanity throughout history and that human beings give different meanings to this involvement. These include the possibility of contact with the sacred and to promote religious experiences; to serve as a method for coping with adverse conditions such as illness or physical or psychological problems; to be used as spices in cooking; to alter consciousness; and for recreational purposes. Considering this variety of functions and the great importance that drugs have for humanity, it is not be surprising that they began to be of economic interest to the capitalist society, resulting in a series of explorations (Carneiro 2005).

Furthermore, the social, cultural, and economic influences of drugs on people's lives resulted in a reaction of control and power over such substances, based on

T. M. Ronzani (✉)
Universidade Federal de Juiz de Fora, Juiz de Fora, Brazil
e-mail: telmo.ronzani@ufjf.edu.br

T. M. Ronzani (ed.), *Drugs and Social Context*,
https://doi.org/10.1007/978-3-319-72446-1_1

ideologies that establish relations of domination and control over specific populations, passing from the moral and religious to legal and criminal discourse and, most recently, to medical discourse. Accordingly, the different functions of drug use are regulated by specific areas that dominate, define, or sell new forms of involvement. According to Escohodato (1998) in his book *History of Drugs*, substance use in society is now governed as a new form of sin, or by codes of conduct that lead to new forms of crime. A third form of social control is by new forms of pathologies and the consequent possibilities of "treatment of addictions."

We know that such factors are closely related to these complex and subtle (sometimes not so subtle) forms of control of individuals or populations. Throughout recent history, the drugs theme was controlled mainly through religion, linking certain substances and their consumption to sinful behavior (Escohodato 1998). Beyond rhetorical control, treatment of dependence was tied to religious sectors or to philanthropy, under strong religious and moral connotations, or as an "entity" concealed within the treatment of "madness" (Pontes 2017). A second approach is related to the legal and juridical aspect that places drug consumption as a crime and, as a result, punishes the people who use drugs (Boiteux et al. 2017).

More recently, the medical paradigm has become dominant, with drug use being seen as unhealthy behavior and, consequently, in the domain of the medical sector, which defines actions on the user-patient. Associated with this aspect, large profits are generated by the pharmaceutical industry, which commercially exploits the therapeutic properties of some psychoactive substances and generates the Manichaean classification of good and bad drugs.

The medical-disease discourse appears in a very legitimating form of moral-religious and criminal-legal reasoning, because it brings with it the status of "scientific," so dear to modern society, and therefore reinforces, through the disease, morally reprehensible and legally criminalized behaviors (Adams 2008). Scientific status has gained even more ideological power with recent neuroscientific discussions that advocate dependence as a "chronic brain disease" (Volkow and Morales 2015). From there, we find biological explanations for this "dysfunction" and can act on these individuals from the medical-pharmacological point of view or even scientifically justify seclusion and isolation for treatment. This creates a very favorable environment for the control of specific groups. That is, if drug use is a disease that affects the individual biologically and, in turn, this individual causes harm to others, the power of decision should lie with specialists in the field, creating mechanisms for punishing users and some drug dealers (Fiore 2005). The situation is then, supposedly, under control.

Obviously, this social construction of perceptions about use and users is part of a historical process and several different models have been generated over time. Table 1.1 shows different models of perception regarding drug use, as proposed by Palm (2006).

Some aspects of these proposed models deserve attention. The first is that the different views are not presented linearly or separately from a historical point of view. That is, they are interrelated and, throughout history, there have been advances or setbacks due to the contextual aspects involved. A second point regards the public health model. Viewing drug use from the public health perspective has been rightly

Table 1.1 Models of perception about alcohol and drug use

Moral model: Use of alcohol and other drugs is a sign of weakness and lack of character, whereas abstinence is seen as a sign of virtue. Dependence is seen by society as a crime and therefore should be treated
Medical or disease model: There is still a remnant of moralization regarding use, but dependence is no longer seen as a moral issue, but rather as a disease. Addiction is perceived as a problem of the individual and not of the drug itself
Rationalist model: Influenced by capitalism, with the normative idea that dependence is the result of a failure in self-control, an irrational act
Public health model: The focus is not the user individually, but the environment and all users and the problems associated with use. Actions are viewed collectively, based on different usage patterns and general health policies. The main concern is to reduce consumption and the overall consequences
Social model: Dependence is seen as a consequence of misery and social injustice, and therefore should be seen as a problem of society

Source: Palm (2006)

defended as a way to overcome the individual, biological, and criminalizing hegemonic view in many countries (Adams 2008). On the other hand, this same model has served as justification for hygienist actions and cleansing of cities and certain social groups, as discussed in more depth in later chapters. Therefore, there must be critical appraisal of the true function of appropriation of drug use as a public health issue (Ronzani et al. 2009; Ronzani 2013).

The social approach to drug use does not necessarily present itself as negative to biological or intersubjective aspects, but draws attention to the need to broaden the discussion on such a complex subject that generates injustice and suffering for certain groups. I call attention to a book by Adams (2008), entitled *Fragmented Intimacy. Addiction in a Social World*, where he states that drug use is essentially social, because we can understand the problem of drug use or addiction mainly in the relationship between one person and another or with his/her group, within a specific context. Adams makes an important contribution by calling attention to the importance of culture and ideologies in understanding the relationship of individuals with the world, especially by demonstrating that this social and cultural aspect contributes to a broader understanding of dependence.

I draw particular attention to the importance of considering social determinants in understanding drug abuse problems. Although drug use is present in several social classes and in different contexts, some determinants increase the social burden of this behavior. That is, there is no simple and direct relationship between cause and effect. Some of these social determinants related to drug use are poverty, race, gender, unemployment, housing, education, and malnutrition (Matsumoto and Gimenez 2017; Wilkinson and Marmot 2003). Emphasis on determinants enables a better understanding of the social vulnerability of substance users, and therefore can optimize action planning and care for users (McCormack et al. 2005; Mota et al. 2014).

Accordingly, in this chapter and more broadly in this book, we expand this spectrum to show that, beyond the importance of understanding the direct interaction between the user and other individuals or groups, there is a macrosocial determination that fundamentally mediates how drug consumption occurs. For example, within the current capitalist society, can we consider that drug use by rich and poor, by black and white, and by people living in different regions with different social situations of vulnerability is the same use or even the same problem? It is important to think beyond the pharmacological properties or means of administration of a given substance. Where, in which historical moment or social context, and by whom a substance is consumed are fundamental for understanding the possible damages associated with use.

Therefore, when we consider the economic and social organization present in the capitalist model, macrosocial aspects have great importance in understanding what drugs mean in our context. Specifically, it is fundamental to understand how our model of the consumer society, the generated profit, and the forms of oppression legitimize the discourse regarding controlling and "combating" drugs. For this, there is nothing better than analyzing the history of drugs to understand their importance for the economic model of society.

1.2 Between Heaven and Hell: The Importance of Drugs as a Market

Since the beginning of mercantilism, that is, since the development of capitalism began, drugs have had a contradictory meaning (Carneiro 2005). On one hand, they were one of the main drivers of the great voyages to set up commercial relations between Europe, the Orient, and the Americas. On the other hand, drugs were also seen as a great "evil" to society. Obviously, we can note from this negative reaction that there were other implicit objectives, as stated by Ecohodato (Escohodato 1998):

> "Infernal substances, heroic medicine, goods for overseas exchange, the drugs of paganism emerge in daylight. Although strictly prohibited as 'travel' vehicles, a statute of doctors, pharmacists and pharmaceutical chemists extends its use in increasingly active preparations. At the same time appeared drugs of extraordinary future, which are received from the beginning with marked ambivalence. Drugs have always been an important means of communication between distant cultures; but from now on it is the continents that export and import them massively, and with it are detected the first germs of xenophobia linked to one or another substance." (Escohodato 1998, p. 261)

Understanding drug use as a *public health problem* is closely linked to the development of capitalism. According to historians, the wealth sought in the Americas and the Orient during the great voyages of the sixteenth and seventeenth centuries was mainly in the form of drugs, either for use as spices or for their psychoactive effects. Therefore, we can say that drugs were the great driver of mercantile and economic relations, bringing with them the exploitation of specific peoples (Carneiro 2005). Social inequalities produced by the accumulation of capital and violence against specific people have a background of invasions, looting, and actions of economic protectionism linked to drugs (Carneiro 2005; Escohodato 1998). The discovery by European settlers of substances with great potential for economic and commercial exploitation led to the violent removal of knowledge about these substances from those regions (Carneiro 2005).

Trade protectionism was the genesis of global prohibitionism, because the incentive for or prohibition of trade, cultivation, and production of some drugs were linked to the commercial interests of certain countries (Escohodato 1998). Since that time, sanctions on the use and trade of certain substances has been linked to deterioration of the identities of certain peoples and ethnic groups, Such sanctions sought to socially justify the ban by linking the inappropriate moral conduct of certain people with the consumption of that substance. Therefore, the stigmatization and deterioration of identities and consequent actions of violence and social injustice were legitimized by production of this sense of subcultures. This practice has been in constant use for a long time and is still common practice.

An illustrative example can be found in the book by Brazilian historians Renato Pinto Venâncio and Henrique Carneiro (2005) that, with other collaborators, discusses how the production of *cachaça*, a spirit made from sugarcane in Brazil, was instrumental in sustaining slavery. It was the main currency of exchange, along with tobacco, in the slave trade between the Americas and Africa. Alcohol, tobacco, and various other psychotropic drugs were therefore the main commercial sources of livelihood in the colonies and one of the principal forms of capital accumulation.

Incidentally, the consumption and trade of *cachaça* in Brazil during this period serves as an example of the ambiguous relationship that many countries have with drugs. On one hand, the production of *cachaça* had great importance for the maintenance of slavery; on the other hand, it generated a problem in the trade balance and for that reason was the subject of political manipulations (Guimarães 2005). The increase in *cachaça* consumption in the colonies, Portugal, and other European countries caused major problems with the commercial expansion of Portuguese wine. Competition between the sale of *cachaça* (low cost, low price, and high consumption among the poorest people) and Portuguese wine became a commercial problem for Portugal. This situation led to prohibition of the production of *cachaça* in Brazil by the Portuguese crown, with the argument that its consumption was linked to black people and the poor, causing social degeneration, and that action was necessary to curb this addiction (Guimarães 2005).

Later, it was realized that production of *cachaça* could be a way to reduce the agricultural crisis in Portugal and that its sale could be exploited in other European countries. Therefore, its production was again allowed and stimulated. In addition, at some point, consumption of *cachaça* was allowed or even encouraged among slaves, because of its powers of diminishing the suffering and pain of their precarious conditions of survival and for the purpose of control over docile slaves (Valadares 2005). Thus, I call attention to the genesis of another element of the social function of promoting drug use, in particular those drugs produced by current pharmaceutical industries: anesthetization and alienation in the face of exploitative relationships established in capitalist society.

This example and others demonstrate that the prohibition or not of a particular drug has much more to do with economic issues and the social groups that consume it than with the potential damage caused, however much they try to convince us otherwise. Another example was the reaction of the United States to the arrival of certain groups of immigrants and their pejorative association with the consumption of drugs, such as the use of marijuana among black people and Latinos and the use of opium among the Chinese who came to work on the construction of railways. These groups were seen as a social threat to white Americans because of prejudice against immigrants and competition for work. Thus, these groups were quickly associated with stereotypes, certain drugs, and disapproved social behaviors such as violence, banditry, and moral deterioration (Escohodato 1998). As a result, there was a reaction in the form of social isolation mechanisms, punishment, and imprisonment legitimized mainly by the prohibited consumption of some drugs (Fiore 2005).

1.3 Drug Use and Forms of Criminality in the Consumer Society

This section discusses more specifically the social factors related to drug use in the recent period, after commercial expansion and the establishment of business between continents and countries. With the advent of the Industrial Revolution, there was also growth in the production and marketing of drugs, which moved to newer forms of production and as a highly profitable business for some countries. Therefore, in the new consumer society, drugs remain a product of great economic interest, encouraged by commercial and industrial agglomerations. The main context of drug use is in the search for pleasure and to reduce the suffering produced by the forms of work imposed on a large proportion of workers.

Over time, large-scale production has a big impact on the consumer society; new drugs are produced and new ways of control, as Escohotado (1998) points out:

> "There are several high-potency psychoactive substances, both in the field of stimulants and sedatives, and because they are not yet attached to marginal groups or colonizable crops, remain as simple medicines. Featuring these drugs without complications, many who usually resorted to natural opiates and cocaine decided—with higher or lower desire—to sedate and stimulate themselves with the new products, which were pure, cheap and almost as effective for the basic needs of peace and energy. From the thirties, the diffusion of this alternative drug offer makes pharmacies have, for the clientele of similar products, as many prepared with as much influence on the mood as at the end of the nineteenth century." (Escohodato 1998, p. 511)

Since then, we have what Carneiro (2005) calls the "fetish goods" model, offering substances with increasingly powerful effects that blend with modern consumerism, where not only goods are bought and sold but also sensations and internal trips. Accordingly, drugs and their effects have a high status in the modern consumer society. Based on the consumer society, the model seeks to deny social and individual discomfort produced by this society and uses various devices to do so, by creating either guilty parties or curtains of smoke that hide or camouflage the inequalities produced by this model of society. In this way, we choose our poisons according to the interests of groups that hold power or even access to consumption; this includes *assigning ethical qualities to chemicals* (Escohodato 1998).

Obviously, within the consumer goods production process and the great economic inequalities produced by this model, there are people who have access to certain products. Mechanisms are even created so that these products remain exclusive to certain groups or representatives of a certain social class. For this, there are well-established strategies of stimulating or punishing behaviors linked to certain social determinants. This control is performed mainly by the State, which sets laws, crimes, and prohibitions that especially affect economically marginalized populations. Control is often linked to certain behaviors against an individual's failure to have jurisdiction or access to certain consumer goods strategically defined as legal, moral, or allowed. In this regard, public policies emerge, influenced by so-called moral entrepreneurs (Escohodato 1998), which define such actions through speeches about health, security, or justice (Fiore 2005).

As a result, we have actions of pathologization, criminalization, or exclusion of certain group's rights, mainly linked to the liberal ideal of failure or individual incompetence in the face of opportunities for access to certain goods and services, geared especially to the poor, specifically black populations and economically peripheral countries.

Cleaning the system of the "side effects of capital accumulation," includes their punishment or removal from the view of this so-called ideal society, where the use of certain drugs among specific groups is related to other social conditions and the mechanisms of poverty and criminalization implemented a while ago:

> "*Then appears (early nineteenth century) the distinction between culpable and non-culpable poverty, advocating the disappearance of the old assistencial care system, because it is understood that generous private charity raises the problem instead of reducing it. As far as possible, marginals should be incorporated into the labor market and, moreover, their care should not take away the energy of those who are fit to work. Faced with the non-segregating solution, the segregator was proposed, and in front of private, was proposed the institutional attention. The proper is to promote the internment of any deviant, understanding for this not only the poor, the diminished and the sick, but also the extravagant ones, the drunks, the orphans, the uprooted adolescents, the crazy ones, the old ones and the set of felons or people who committed faults not punished with death, torture or pillory. For the bums are reformed the English workhouses, with much harder systems of treatment, and for the other was inaugurated reformatories, asylums and public nursing homes.*" (Escohodato 1998, p. 374)

This whole context of producing meaning for the consumption of certain drugs and their specific linkage was an important basis for the implementation of various geopolitical strategies, coincidentally or not at a time when the world was under military control and expansion to strategic territories desirable. At that time, the "drug war" discourse within the context of international relations justified the military invasion of several countries, drawing special attention to Latin America and forging the idea of producer and consumer countries. In general, producing countries coincide with those of the southern hemisphere and consumers with those of the northern hemisphere. The proposed way to fight this war was to attack the production zones and establish military bases in those regions, with the support of international organizations. This had several results, including the expulsion of peasants from their lands, militarization of certain regions, and pauperization of communities. However, there was no decrease in drug consumption, but instead an increase in corruption linked to trafficking, social marginalization, paramilitary groups strengthened by recruiting the poorest people, and increasing violence in those regions (Fiore 2005). In other words, it was a failed war against drugs, but perhaps a powerful and victorious strategy of control, exploitation, and maintenance of the *status quo*. In this respect, it is important to emphasize that "a drug is not only a certain chemical compound, but something whose effects depend on the conditions for access to it" (Escohodato 1998, p. 492). I would add that knowledge of the macrosocial conditions related to drug use is fundamental for deepening understanding of this issue.

1.4 Us and Them: Social Construction of Legitimizing of Inequality Production Processes

As already discussed, any social construction based on the choice of encouraging or prohibiting certain drugs is rooted in socioeconomic and political processes that purposely target certain behaviors and lead to processes of stigmatization and discrimination. It is no coincidence, for example, that the consumption of alcoholic beverages in certain contexts is highly encouraged and socially approved. In addition, drugs marketed by large pharmaceutical conglomerates are increasingly posed as the solution for problems such as depression, stress, irritability, and fatigue (Dalla Vecchia et al. 2017). In another direction, we observe the perception of crack users and crack use as aberrations and causes of social ills, giving the user the status of subhuman and linked to poverty, the street context, and individual failure (Silveira et al. 2016).

Brazil is one of the clearest examples of policies that still segregate and punish groups marginalized in its history. Data from the National Survey of Penitentiary Information (Brasil 2016) demonstrate that the prison population of Brazil has been increasing every year, today being the fourth largest in the world. Of those in prison, 46% are there from the enforcement of drug laws. The people incarcerated in Brazil for drug trafficking are characterized mainly by the fact that they are mostly black, from socioeconomically low classes, small traffickers, with no criminal record, and not carrying a weapon at the time of arrest. The punishment linked to the use of drugs has a strong class and racial bias that has been historically present in Brazil since the time of slavery, when black people received different punishment from white people (Petuco 2016). Even post-abolition, the penal code included specific punishments for "drunkards, bums, and *capoeiras*" (Pontes 2017).

The organization of the consumer society establishes classifications or social rules, especially with the prospect of separation between "us," with access to consumer goods, and "them," the subcitizens that cannot consume goods because of individual incompetence and therefore must be separated from the so-called good citizens. Through norms and social rules defined by dominant groups, it is stipulated that deviations from such norms are subject to social control and punishment legitimized by the State (the direct representative of such dominant groups) (Becker 2008).

In this sense, specific drugs related to "second class" people in society are strongly stigmatized, which justifies processes of marginalization of specific social groups and the moralization, punishment, and violation of human rights of these subcitizens (Levin and van Laar 2004; Silveira et al. 2013).

Furthermore, I call attention to a perspective that at first can be seen as positive: the liberal-progressive view of drug use, which defends individual freedoms and decisions based on the needs and desires of the people. This view is already a major advance if we consider the history and current scenarios of repression and criminalization of drug use. However, it is important to emphasize that we must go further and also consider that macrosocial aspects and their determination are of paramount importance in understanding the policies, culture, and even the impacts of drug use in the world and how this theme is directly related to the production of social injustice. This discussion has been held in more detail in another text (Dalla Vecchia et al. 2017), but it is important to emphasize the possible trap posed by automatically linking the ideals of individual liberalism with economic liberalism. In the latter, the market becomes the regulator of drug marketing and an indicator of access to social rights (according to the idea of the citizen-consumer), with the danger of reinforcing the idea of rights for those who have access to their use.

1.5 Final Considerations

As we have seen, the way we perceive drug use is related to historical and cultural processes. It is quite common to find in several sources of information an idea of what is meant by the problem of drug use or even a straightforward conclusion that social ills, whether violence, unemployment, corruption, hunger, or poor school or work performance, are directly caused by drugs. We have the temptation, sometimes well-intentioned and sometimes not, to find magical or simplistic solutions to these problems. In this sense, I argue that we are doubly mistaken. First, as we have seen, drug use itself is not the problem, but rather the way that society uses that substance (or commodity). The second misconception is that by defining a place in the body for such a "disease," we can find the solution; as already argued, there are much broader factors involved in this issue.

It is not intended to deny the potential problems that drug use can cause for some people, whether biological, psychological, or social. I argue the need for a more integrative and dynamic view when considering that medium or macrosocial factors are important for understanding the individual impacts. Moreover, the impact of substance use is mediated by various social determinants in different ways.

Finally, the main point I would like to make is that drugs are just another component that have been inserted, among many others, into this consumer society and that the meanings produced by this often serve as mechanisms of control and maintenance of legitimized situations of social inequality between social groups and countries. If we do not look at this and the model of society we have produced, we can only have a minimally approximate reflection or action regarding the issue.

References

Adams, P. J. (2008). *Fragmented intimacy. Addiction in social world.* New York: Springer.

Becker, H. S. (2008). *Outsiders. Estudo de Sociologia do Desvio.* Rio de Janeiro: Zahar.

Boiteux, L., Chernicharo, L. P., & Alves, C. S. (2017). Direitos humanos e convenções internacionais de drogas: Em busca de uma razão humanitária nas leis de drogas. In: Dalla Vecchia, M., Ronzani, T. M., Paiva, F. S., Batista, C. B., & Costa, P. H. A. (Orgs.). *Drogas e Direitos Humanos: Reflexões em Tempos de Guerra às Drogas* (pp. 233-264). Porto Alegre: Rede Unida.

Brasil (Ministério da Justiça). (2016). *Levantamento Nacional de Informações Penitenciárias INFOPEN.* Brasil: Ministério da Justiça.

Carneiro, H. (2005). Tranformações do significado da palavra "droga": das especiarias coloniais ao proibicionismo contemporâneo. In R. P. Venâncio & H. Carneiro (Eds.), *Álcool e drogas na história do Brasil* (pp. 11–28). Belo Horizonte: Editora PUC-Minas.

Dalla Vecchia, M., Ronzani, T. M., & Azevedo, B. L. (2017). Os Cuidados à Saúde dos Usuários de Drogas em Perspectiva Psicossocial: Conquistas e Desafios 10 Anos após a Nova Lei de Drogas. In ABRAPSO (Ed.), *Democracia, Política e Psicologia Social: Rupturas e Consolidações (pp. 168-181).* Porto Alegre: ABRAPSO.

Escohodato, A. (1998). *Historia natural de las drogas* (7th ed.). Madrid: Alianza Editorial.

Fiore, M. (2005). A medicalização da questão do uso de drogas no Brasil: reflexões acerca de debates institucionais e jurídicos. In: Venâncio, R.P. and Carneiro, H (Orgs.). *Álcool e drogas história do Brasil* (pp. 257-290). Belo Horizonte: Editora PUC-Minas.

Guimarães, C.M. (2005). Os quilombos a noite e a aguardente nas Minas coloniais. In: Venâncio, R.P., & Carneiro, H (orgs). *Álcool e drogas história do Brasil* (pp. 93-122). Belo Horizonte: Editora PUC-Minas.

Levin, S., & van Laar, C. (2004). *Stigma and group inequality. Social psychological perspectives.* New York: Psychology Press.

Matsumoto, A. E., & Gimenez, S. G. (2017). Sistema carcerário e criminologia crítica. In: Dalla Vecchia, M., Ronzani, T. M., Paiva, F. S., Batista, C. B., & Costa, P. H. A. (Orgs.). *Drogas e Direitos Humanos: Reflexões em Tempos de Guerra às Drogas* (pp. 265–287). Porto Alegre: Rede Unida.

McCormack, R. P., Hoffman, L. F., Norman, M., Goldfrank, L. R., & Norman, E. M. (2005). Voices of homeless alcoholics who frequent Bellevue hospital: A qualitative study. *Annals of Emergency Medicine, 65*(2), 178–186.

Mota, D.C.B., Ronzani, T.M., & Moura, Y.G. (2014). Tratamento e apoio psicossocial às pessoas em situação de rua usuárias de drogas. In: Grinover, A.P., Assagra G, Gustin M, Lima PCV, Lenaco R (orgs.). *Direitos Fundamentais das Pessoas em Situação de Rua* (pp. 497–514). Belo Horizonte: D'Plácido.

Palm, J. (2006). *Moral concerns: treatment staff and users perspectives on alcohol and other problems* (PhD. thesis). Stockholm: University of Stockholm.

Petuco, D.R.S. (2016). *O Pomo da Discórdia? A constituição de um campo de lutas em torno das políticas públicas e das técnicas de cuidado em saúde dirigidas a pessoas que usam álcool e outras drogas no Brasil.* (Ph.D. Thesis). Juiz de Fora: Universidade Federal de Juiz de Fora (UFJF).

Pontes, A. K. (2017). *Subjetividades desviantes e políticas de internação: ébrios habituais e alcoolistas no Rio de Janeiro durante a Primeira República* (1899-1920). (Ph.D. thesis). Rio de Janeiro: Universidade Federal do Rio de Janeiro (UFRJ).

Ronzani, T. M. (2013). *Ações Integradas Sobre Drogas. Prevenção, Abordagens e Políticas Públicas.* Juiz de Fora: Editora UFJF.

Ronzani, T. M., Furtado, E. F., & Higgins-Biddle, J. (2009). Stigmatization of alcohol and other drug users by primary care providers in Southeast Brazil. *Social Science & Medicine, 69*(7), 1080–1084.

Silveira, P. S., Casela, A. L. M., Monteiro, E. P., Freitas, J. V. T., & Machado, N. M. (2016). Vulnerabilidade, estigma e uso de drogas. In F. Garcia, M. R. Costa, L. P. Guimarães, & M. C. L. Neves (Eds.), *Vulnerabilidade e Uso de Drogas* (pp. 37–48). Belo Horizonte: Editora PUC-Minas.

Silveira, P. S., Soares, R. G., Noto, A. R., & Ronzani, T. M. (2013). Estigma e suas consequências para usuários de drogas. In: Ronzani, T. M. (Org.). *Ações Integradas Sobre Drogas. Prevenção, Abordagens e Políticas Públicas* (pp. 248–274). Juiz de Fora: Ed. UFJF.

Valadares, V. (2005). O consumo de aguardente em Minas Gerais no final do século XVIII: uma visão entre os poderes metropolitanos e colonial. In: Venâncio, R.P., & Carneiro, H. (orgs). *Álcool e drogas história do Brasil* (pp. 123–140). Belo Horizonte: Editora PUC-Minas.

Venâncio, R. P., & Carneiro, H. (2005). *Álcool e drogas história do Brasil*. Belo Horizonte: Editora PUC-Minas.

Volkow, N. D., & Morales, M. (2015). The brain on drugs: From reward to addiction. *Cell, 162*(4), 712–725.

Wilkinson, R., & Marmot, M. (2003). *Social determinants of health: The solid facts*. Geneva: WHO.

Chapter 2
The Stigmatization of Drug Use as Mechanism of Legitimation of Exclusion

Pollyanna Santos da Silveira, Joanna Gonçalves Andrade de Tostes, Hoi Ting Wan, Telmo Mota Ronzani, and Patrick W. Corrigan

Abstract Drug abuse is considered one of the most stigmatizing health conditions. Growing evidence has shown that stigma is associated with the different impairments of stigmatized individuals. The impacts of social stigma include insufficient access to health care, worse indicators of education and employment and, consequently, a negative effect on income. Regarding the availability of services, many people who could benefit from health care do not receive it. In this sense, social stigma becomes a barrier in the search for help and in adherence to treatment. On the other hand, moralizing strategies associated with prohibitionist perspectives, besides being ineffective, restrict the possibilities of access to care for people with problems related to the use of drugs. The lack of trust in treatment services and their efficacy, in addition to stigmatization, has been identified as an important barrier to treatment. This problem requires changes in the screening, detection, and referral of treatment for addiction. Thus, overcoming stigma is necessary to ensure that evidence-based strategies and indicators of effectiveness are used.

2.1 Concept of Social Stigma

Modern conceptualizations of stigma as social injustice can be traced to Erving Goffman (1963), who framed stigma as a mark that leads to "spoiled identity." He believed stigma of all kinds (related to ethnicity, gender, sexual orientation, age, and illness) to be an attribute that is socially discrediting, causing people to being unjustly

P. S. da Silveira
Universidade Católica de Petrópolis, Petrópolis, Brazil
e-mail: pollyannassilveira@gmail.com

J. G. A. de Tostes · T. M. Ronzani (✉)
Universidade Federal de Juiz de Fora, Juiz de Fora, Brazil
e-mail: joanna@tostes.org; tm.ronzani@gmail.com

H. T. Wan · P. W. Corrigan
Illinois Institute of Technology, Chicago, IL, USA
e-mail: cheryl_281230@yahoo.com.hk; corrigan@iit.edu

T. M. Ronzani (ed.), *Drugs and Social Context*,
https://doi.org/10.1007/978-3-319-72446-1_2

Table 2.1 Matrix describing the stigma of substance use disorders (SUDs)

		Types		
		Public	Self	Label avoidance
Social cognitive structures	Stereotypes and prejudice	*People with SUDs are immoral, to blame for their disorder, and criminal*	*I am dangerous, immoral, and to blame. Leads to lowered self-esteem and self-efficacy*	*I perceive that the public disrespects and discriminates against people with substance use disorders*
	Discrimination	*Employers do not hire them, landlords do not rent to them, and primary care providers offer a worse standard of care*	*Why try? Someone like me is unworthy or unable to work, live independently, or have good health*	*I do not want this. I will avoid the label by not seeking out treatment*

Examples are provided in each of the cells

rejected. Corrigan et al. (2016a, b) developed a matrix useful for understanding the stigma of disease in general, and addictions more specifically. The matrix (see Table 2.1) is defined by two dimensions: social cognitive structures that underlie stigma and types of stigma that meaningfully impact a person with illness.

2.1.1 Stereotypes

Social psychologists distinguish between the largely private experience of stigma in general (stereotyping and prejudice) from the more public, behavioral result that is discrimination (Crocker et al. 1998). Stereotypes are harmful and disrespectful beliefs about a group. What stereotypes might be candidates for the foundation of addiction stigma? Schomerus et al. (2011) began to establish a content-valid measure of alcohol stigma. To identify the stereotypes of alcohol addiction, they conducted focus groups consisting of people with alcohol dependence, providers, and family members. They generated 16 stereotype candidates, including "unreliable," "emotionally unstable," "living at other's expense," and "self-pitying." A similar set of qualitative interviews were conducted to identify candidate stereotypes of "drug users" (Radcliffe and Stevens 2008). Although the resulting analysis from the latter study yielded compelling themes about the form of stigma, specific stereotypes per se did not emerge from their work.

How is a stereotype distinguished from accurate perception? For example, research seems to suggest that violence and crime are associated with drug misuse, although this is a complex relationship with full description requiring additional constructs such as the social determinants of illegal activity (Bennett et al. 2008). Might stereotypes reflect a kernel of truth, that, for example, people who use drugs are in fact dangerous (Allport 1979)? The kernel of truth rests on assumptions about stereotype accuracy (e.g., research supports the stereotype that "basketball players are tall"). Mostly dated science uses this rationale to argue for accuracy in trait impressions of ethnic groups, such as the Irish are drawn to alcohol or Asians are mathematically strong (Abate and Berrien 1967). Currently, social psychologists are skeptical about the notion of kernel of truth and stereotype accuracy, recognizing that social science is incapable of defining the "traits" of a group in this way (Jost and Banaji 1994). History is replete with assertions that are racist in the guise of kernel of truth. For example, some have asserted that African Americans are intellectually inferior on the basis of population data representing IQ tests (Jensen 1969) when, in fact, better constructed research suggests that any differences in existing scholastic tests represent stereotype threat and concomitant evaluation anxiety (Steele and Aronson 1995). In terms of social policy, any theory that suggests legitimacy of stigma can egregiously be used to further justify discrimination against a group.

2.1.2 Prejudice and Discrimination

Stereotypes are unavoidable; they are learned as part of growing up in a culture; for example, American children learn at a young age that "addicts" are dangerous (Corrigan and Watson 2002). Being prejudiced is agreeing with the stereotype, leading to emotional and evaluative consequences: "That's right! All those addicts are violent and I fear them." In path models, affective responses to stereotypes (another element of prejudice) are often mediators between stereotypes and its behavioral result, discrimination: "And because I *fear* addicts, I will not hire them, rent to them, give them the same opportunities at school, or let them worship with my congregation."

Three emotional responses mediate stereotyping and subsequent discriminatory behavior (Corrigan et al. 2003; Pingani et al. 2012): (1) fear, causing unfair discrimination that undermines personal goals related to work, independent living, relationships, and health; (2) blame (believing people caused their addiction), leading to anger and subsequently to discrimination, often in the guise of unnecessarily coercive treatments; and (3) internalized blame (I caused my addiction because I am weak), leading to shame (decreased sense of self-esteem and self-efficacy).

2.1.3 Stigma Types

Discrimination's impact becomes clear when realizing it varies by type (Corrigan and Kosyluk 2014; Phelan et al. 2008). Three types are summarized in Table 2.1: public stigma, label avoidance, and self-stigma.

Public stigma occurs when the general population endorses stereotypes and decides to discriminate against people labeled as "addicts." Research shows that employers are less likely to hire and landlords are less likely to rent to people with substance use disorders (SUDs) (van Olphen et al. 2009; Spencer et al. 2008). There is also discrimination when seeking public office or pursuing work in child care (van Boekel et al. 2013). Research shows that health care providers admit to the stigma of addiction (Henderson et al. 2008), which leads to withholding primary care (Weiss et al. 2004) and pharmacy services to people with addictions that are in need (Anstice et al. 2009).

Stigma is likely to undermine support for harm reduction strategies such as safe injection facilities and needle exchange programs (Rivera et al. 2014). However, this is a complex relationship, with the impact of addiction stigma conflated with criminalization. For example, research shows that people who endorse the depth of legal penalties for substance use agree with greater discrimination against people with SUDs (West et al. 2014). Future research needs to unpack the relative impact of addiction and criminalization stigma as well as the ways they interact.

Public stigma impacts care seeking for people with SUD when it leads to *label avoidance*. Epidemiological research shows that only 25% of people with SUDs ever participate in any care program (Dawson et al. 2005). People who perceive higher stigma toward peers with SUDs are less likely to use treatment programs for alcoholism (Keyes et al. 2010) and less likely to participate in sterile syringe programs (Rivera et al. 2014). These are mostly small and compartmentalized studies; however, future research needs to tackle these questions more broadly and rigorously.

Self-stigma occurs when people with mental illness internalize the corresponding prejudice (Link 1987; Link et al. 2001). A regressive model of self-stigma has four stages (Corrigan and Watson 2002), in which people are (1) aware of the stigma of mental illness (also called perceived stigma: "The public thinks people with substance use disorders are dangerous" [Phelan et al. 2000]), which might lead to (2) agreeing with the stigma ("Yep; that's right. Addicts are dangerous!"), followed by (3) self-application ("I'm an addict so I must be dangerous"), which (4) negatively impacts self-esteem ("I am less of a person because I am an addict and dangerous") and self-efficacy ("I am less able to accomplish my goals because I am mentally ill and dangerous"). Self-discrimination causes the "why try effect" (Corrigan et al. 2016): "Why try to seek a job; someone like me is not worthy." "Why try to live independently; someone like me is not able."

Self-stigma seems to have an equally egregious effect on the well-being of people with addictions (Luoma et al. 2013). Research by Schomerus et al. (2011) partially validated the regressive model of self-stigma for people with alcohol dependence. Namely, people who apply stereotypes to themselves report greater harm to self-esteem, which, in turn, seems to undermine drink-refusal self-efficacy. Other studies showed self-stigma of addictions to be associated with greater depression and anxiety, as well as diminished psychological well-being (Brown et al. 2015; Luoma et al. 2013). Interestingly, some research suggests that self-stigma does not always lead to harmful effects. One study showed that people with higher self-stigma were more likely to stay in treatment longer, leading to higher abstinence (Luoma et al. 2014). This finding shows the complexity of stigma in addiction, calling for research that looks at the varied directions of, in this case, self-stigma on the person who internalizes stereotypes.

2.2 Moralization of Drug Use and Consequences of Stigmatization

2.2.1 Stigma and Substance Use Disorders

Drug abuse is one of the most serious public health problems in the world, and the prevalence of users has been growing over the years. These problems, although largely avoidable, represent a significant social and health burden globally (WHO 2016). Drug abuse is also one of the most stigmatized conditions, even compared with stigmatized mental illnesses. There is a consensus among specialists, advocates, and stakeholders that the stigma of addiction has a negative effect on clinical outcomes and the well-being of people with SUDs or those who are users but do not have a disorder (Corrigan et al. 2016a, b).

Studies have shown that alcohol and drug addiction are one of most stigmatized condition (Silveira et al. 2015), being judged as much more responsible for their condition. In addition, substance addicts cause more social rejection and more negative emotions in the general population and are at particular risk of social and structural discrimination (Schomerus et al. 2011).

The intense rejection of drug dependence is closely related to the way society has been dealing with the issues that are associated with it, ranging from explanatory models to social practices guided by them. Throughout history, conceptual definitions related to drug addiction have characteristics that tend to moralize behaviors and problems that occur as a result of substance abuse. The moderate consensus among the theoretical models that try to explain it makes this condition capable of producing several negative reactions. Among them, shame, rejection, and guilt stand out; these reactions end up ignoring the social and biological context of addicts (Frank and Nagel 2017).

The reasons why drug users are subject to stigma are diverse and complex, involving historical, sociopolitical, and economic factors. However, it is necessary to recognize how current attitudes and public policies reflect the dominant moral model of addiction in the first half of the twentieth century. This model understands that the use of drugs is a personal choice and adopts a critical moral position against this choice. Drug addicts, in this model, are considered weak, antisocial, selfish, lazy, and as people who value pleasure (Pickard 2017).

The medical or disease model makes different assumptions from the moral model, although also widely diffused, and considers dependence a compulsion, a chronic neurobiological disease in which the individual has no rational control or judgment (Frank and Nagel 2017; Pickard 2017). Based on genetic, neurophysiological, neuroscience, and animal models, the medical model has spread the understanding of dependence as a type of "kidnapping of the brain" (Frank and Nagel 2017). To prevent drug addicts from being seen as bad people, and therefore to avoid stigmatization, it is proposed that they should be seen as victims of a chronic and recurrent brain disease and treated with an individual and often decontextualized approach (Heather 2017). However, considering drug addiction as a disease through the adoption of medical terms does not necessarily result in a discourse free of moralization (Frank and Nagel 2017).

Studies have pointed out that substance abuse is also stigmatized by health professionals (Silveira et al. 2015; Ronzani et al. 2009). According to Room et al. (2001), social disapproval of addiction is greater than social disapproval of a range of highly stigmatized conditions, including leprosy, HIV-positive status, homelessness, dirtiness, neglect of children, and a criminal record for burglary. Pickard (2017) emphasizes that stigmatization can be a mark of social disgrace. It carries condemnation and ostracization by society and, typically, creates corresponding shame and isolation on the part of the stigmatized person.

2.2.2 *Consequences of Stigmatization among People with Substance Use Disorders*

The impacts of social stigma include insufficient access to mental health care (Corrigan et al. 2014), reduction in life expectancy, low education levels, unemployment (Silveira et al. 2016), increased risk of connections with criminal justice systems, and poverty (Gronholm et al. 2017). Despite the availability of evidence-based services, epidemiological research suggests that many people who could benefit from health care do not receive it. Thus, social stigma becomes a significant barrier in the search for help (Corrigan et al. 2014).

Substance users might choose to hide their habit or even isolate themselves from social interactions, which could exacerbate the effects of stigma and discrimination (Luoma et al. 2013). Furthermore, substance users may internalize the negative views of society about their health condition, which, in addition to affecting their willingness to seek help and adhere to treatment, can generate negative emotions such as a perception of self-discredit and feelings of worthlessness and devaluation (Li et al. 2009).

The effects of stigma internalization are related to several factors, from the restriction of good life opportunities to difficulty in accessing health services, thereby enhancing the social exclusion of individuals (Li et al. 2009). Studies show that internalized stigma is associated with global impacts on the life of the bearer of a stigmatizing condition, including loss of self-esteem and self-efficacy, which reduce their already limited prospects of recovery. Similarly, individuals who internalize stigma may not adhere to psychiatric treatment in an effort to minimize the chance of being labeled or prevent their condition from being discovered. Some feel hopeless and believe that treatment no longer has an effect on them (Fung et al. 2007; Silveira et al. 2016).

In addition, the negative way that health professionals perceive the user creates obstacles for those seeking treatment, which contributes to their exclusion (Ssebunnya et al. 2009). This leads to poor adherence to treatment, aggravation of symptoms, decrease in quality of life, low self-esteem, and low self-efficacy (Li et al. 2009; Ssebunnya et al. 2009).

As discussed earlier, the impacts of stigma relating to drug use suggest that many people decide not to look for health services or abandon treatment prematurely. Despite the advances in mental health care, studies show that professionals sometimes perform treatment using what could be perceived as coercive means, including hospitalization and reducing an individual's personal control (Corrigan et al. 2014), which is particularly frequent when it comes to users of alcohol and other drugs.

2.3 Stigma, Social Exclusion, and Public Policies: How Stigmatization Becomes Official Exclusion Actions

In the health field, healthcare is inextricably related to public policies, guidelines, and social norms. Accordingly, some questions may be raised, taking into account that health can be conceived as the total or partial realization of separate well-being projects. Going further, the environment in which individuals live influences them, according to their gender, social class, ethnicity, sexuality, and others factors (Gulliford et al. 2013). However, stigma directed at some minority groups and related to certain health conditions is one of the most significant barriers to achieving health (Hatzenbuehler et al. 2013).

Some of the inequalities represented by barriers at the system level are attributed to structural stigma, a macrosocial process that reflects public policies and private institution initiatives that intentionally or unintentionally restrict the opportunities of people with mental disorders (Corrigan et al. 2004). Intentional actions include those that restrict civil rights, occurring in part because of the stigmatizing belief that people with mental disorders are not capable. The unintended manifestations of stigma are related to distribution of resources. As a result of the moralization of substance abuse, for example, the idea that people are responsible for their condition makes it less likely that the government makes the distribution of resources a priority. At the macro-level, structural stigma is related to unequal distribution of resources for mental health. Similarly, not only the provision of services is affected but also the resources for research. Despite the great impact of mental disorders, resources are not available at levels comparable to those distributed for many physical illnesses (Link 1987; Link et al. 2001; Corrigan et al. 2014).

Social stigma has several implications for substance abuse treatment, once professionals are more willing to give poor and coercive treatment. Attached to this, the process of stigmatization reinforces the exclusion model that secures another aspect of discrimination, compulsory treatment. Compulsory treatment is becoming popular in relation to drug use and involves the exercise of power by placing labeled individuals in separate circumstances and treating them differently. This has several implications regarding social relationships and integration impairment, and may also compromise chances for recovery (Schomerus et al. 2011).

As described above, when considering the use of drugs as a choice, the moral model of addiction gives addicts the responsibility of being in their situation and makes them worthy of stigma and the austere treatment that they receive. Hence, as long as the moral model continues to influence conceptions of drug use, implicitly or explicitly, the prejudice and injustices to which drug users are subject may seem justifiable (Pickard 2017). In this context, there is a strong public appeal that considers the brain disease model of addiction as the only way in which the general population, the creators of opinion, and public policy makers can be persuaded not to blame or punish dependent users for their problematic behavior. In other words, rejecting the medical model means believing and spreading the idea that dependency is a moral failure of people with this diagnosis. The main consequence of this argument is the direct opposition: dependence is either a brain disease or a moral failure, which limits understanding the problem in alternative ways (Heather 2017).

Stigmatizing views about drug users legitimize ineffective approaches that not only attribute to users the responsibility for the problems they face, but also blame them for social problems such as violence. Consequently, these stigmatizing views are barriers to the search for treatment and employment, which are important aspects in the recovery and social reintegration of individuals. Overcoming this social stigma is necessary to ensure strategies for prevention, treatment, and social reintegration that focus on the evidence of effectiveness. Furthermore, the involvement of patients in the treatment decision-making process is important, as is considering other requirements of the individual, rather than exclusive focus on abstinence from drug use (Silveira et al. 2016).

2.4 Final Considerations

Corrigan et al. (2016a, b) suggest that studies on stigma related to drug dependence are still limited, predominantly descriptive, and require greater conceptual and empirical sophistication, especially compared with literature on stigma related to mental disorders. However, existing evidence on this topic indicates, according to Grant (1997), that substance dependence brings several negative consequences to individuals, ranging from health consequences to social disabilities. Users are prevented from performing many social roles and are limited to the condition of addiction.

Negative social reactions, based on erroneous or distorted perceptions, may also be harmful. Evidence in the literature indicates that lack of confidence in treatment services and in their effectiveness, as well as stigmatization, are important barriers to the pursuit of treatment. Therefore, changes in the screening and detection methods and in the referral patterns of addiction treatment services are necessary (Grant 1997). As a consequence, many patients who might benefit from treatment do not seek it, as a strategy to avoid stigmatization.

A key duty for all those who are involved in this field is to consolidate countries' abilities to face drug-related public health challenges and offer technical support.

Public health measures must be adequately prioritized, otherwise drug-related mortality, disability, morbidity, and impact on people's well-being will remain a huge global public health problem (WHO 2016).

References

Abate, M., & Berrien, F. K. (1967). Validation of stereotypes: Japanese versus American students. *Journal of Personality and Social Psychology, 7*(4p1), 435.

Allport, G. W. (1979). *The nature of prejudice*. Cambridge, MA: Basic Books.

Anstice, S., Strike, C. J., & Brands, B. (2009). Supervised methadone consumption: Client issues and stigma. *Substance Use & Misuse, 44*(6), 794–808.

Bennett, T., Holloway, K., & Farrington, D. (2008). The statistical association between drug misuse and crime: A meta-analysis. *Aggression and Violent Behavior, 13*(2), 107–118.

Brown, S. A., Kramer, K., Lewno, B., Dumas, L., Sacchetti, G., & Powell, E. (2015). Correlates of self-stigma among individuals with substance use problems. *International Journal of Mental Health and Addiction, 13*(6), 687–698.

Corrigan, P. W., Bink, A. B., Schmidt, A., Jones, N., & Rüsch, N. (2016). What is the impact of self-stigma? Loss of self-respect and the "why try" effect. *Journal of Mental Health, 25*(1), 10–15.

Corrigan, P. W., Druss, B. G., & Perlick, D. A. (2014). The impact of mental illness stigma on seeking and participating in mental health care. *Psychological Science in the Public Interest, 15*(2), 37–70.

Corrigan, P. W., & Kosyluk, K. A. (2014). Mental illness stigma: Types, constructs, and vehicles for change. In P. W. Corrigan (Ed.), *The stigma of disease and disability* (pp. 35–56). Washington, DC: American Psychological Association.

Corrigan, P. W., Markowitz, F. E., & Watson, A. C. (2004). Structural levels of mental illness stigma and discrimination. *Schizophrenia Bulletin, 30*(3), 481–491.

Corrigan, P., Markowitz, F. E., Watson, A., Rowan, D., & Kubiak, M. A. (2003). An attribution model of public discrimination towards persons with mental illness. *Journal of Health and Social Behavior, 44*, 162–179.

Corrigan, P. W., Schomerus, G., Shuman, V., Kraus, D., Perlick, D., Harnish, A., Kulesza, M., Kane-Willis, K., Qin, S., & Smelson, D. (2016a). Developing a research agenda for understanding the stigma of addictions. Part I: Lessons from the mental health stigma literature. *American Journal on Addictions, 26*, 59–66.

Corrigan, P. W., Schomerus, G., Shuman, V., Kraus, D., Perlick, D., Harnish, A., Kulesza, M., Kane-Willis, K., Qin, S., & Smelson, D. (2016b). Developing a research agenda for reducing the stigma of addictions. Part II: Lessons from the mental health stigma literature. *American Journal on Addictions, 26*, 67–74.

Corrigan, P. W., & Watson, A. C. (2002). Understanding the impact of stigma on people with mental illness. *World Psychiatry, 1*(1), 16.

Crocker, J., Major, B., & Steele, C. (1998). Social stigma. In: D. T. Gilbert, S. T. Fiske, & G. Lindzey (Eds.), *The handbook of social psychology* 4th ed., Vol. II, pp. 504–553. Boston: McGraw Hill.

Dawson, D. A., Grant, B. F., Stinson, F. S., Chou, P. S., Huang, B., & Ruan, W. (2005). Recovery from DSM-IV alcohol dependence: United States, 2001–2002. Addiction, 100(3), 281–292.

Frank, L. E., & Nagel, S. K. (2017). Addiction and moralization: The role of the underlying model of addiction. *Neuroethics, 10*, 129–139.

Fung, K. M., Tsang, H. W., Corrigan, P. W., Lam, C. S., & Cheng, W. M. (2007). Measuring self-stigma of mental illness in China and its implications for recovery. *International Journal of Social Psychiatry, 53*, 408–418.

Goffman, E. (1963). *Stigma: Notes on a spoiled identity*. New York: Simon & Schuster.
Grant, B. F. (1997). Barriers to alcoholism treatment: Reasons for not seeking treatment in a general population sample. *Journal of Studies on Alcohol and Drugs, 58*(4), 365–371.
Gronholm, P. C., Henderson, C., Deb, T., & Thornicroft, G. (2017). Interventions to reduce discrimination and stigma: The state of the art. *Social Psychiatry and Psychiatric Epidemiology, 52*, 249–258.
Gulliford, M, Figueiroa-Munoz, J, & Morgan, M. (2013). Meaning of access in health care. In: M. Gulliford, & M. Morgan (Eds.), *Access to health care*. Danvers, MA: Routledge.
Hatzenbuehler, M. L., Phelan, J. C., & Link, B. G. (2013). Stigma as a fundamental cause of population health inequalities. *American Journal of Public Health, 103*, 813–821.
Heather, N. (2017). Q: Is addiction a brain disease or a moral failing? A: Neither. *Neuroethics, 10*, 115–124. https://doi.org/10.1007/s12152-016-9289-0.
Henderson, S., Stacey, C. L., & Dohan, D. (2008). Social stigma and the dilemmas of providing care to substance users in a safety-net emergency department. *Journal of Health Care for the Poor and Underserved, 19*(4), 1336–1349.
Jensen, A. (1969). How much can we boost IQ and scholastic achievement. *Harvard Educational Review, 39*(1), 1–123.
Jost, J. T., & Banaji, M. R. (1994). The role of stereotyping in system-justification and the production of false consciousness. *British Journal of Social Psychology, 33*(1), 1–27.
Keyes, K. M., Hatzenbuehler, M. L., McLaughlin, K. A., Link, B., Olfson, M., Grant, B. F., & Hasin, D. (2010). Stigma and treatment for alcohol disorders in the United States. *American Journal of Epidemiology, 172*(12), 1364–1372.
Li, L., Lee, S. J., Thammawijaya, P., Jiraphongsa, C., & Rotheram-Borus, M. J. (2009). Stigma, social support, and depression among people living with HIV in Thailand. *AIDS Care, 21*(8), 1007–1013.
Link, B. G. (1987). Understanding labeling effects in the area of mental disorders: An assessment of the effects of expectations of rejection. *American Sociological Review, 52*, 96–112.
Link, B. G., Struening, E. L., Neese-Todd, S., Asmussen, S., & Phelan, J. C. (2001). Stigma as a barrier to recovery: The consequences of stigma for the self-esteem of people with mental illnesses. *Psychiatric Services, 52*(12), 1621–1626.
Luoma, J. B., Kulesza, M., Hayes, S. C., Kohlenberg, B., & Larimer, M. (2014). Stigma predicts residential treatment length for substance use disorder. *The American Journal of Drug and Alcohol Abuse, 40*(3), 206–212.
Luoma, J. B., Nobles, R. H., Drake, C. E., Hayes, S. C., O'Hair, A., Fletcher, L., & Kohlenberg, B. S. (2013). Self-stigma in substance abuse: Development of a new measure. *Journal of Psychopathology and Behavioral Assessment, 35*(2), 223–234.
Pickard, H. (2017). Responsibility without blame for addiction. *Neuroethics, 10*, 169–180.
Phelan, J. C., Link, B. G., & Dovidio, J. F. (2008). Stigma and prejudice: One animal or two? *Social Science & Medicine, 67*(3), 358–367.
Phelan, J. C., Link, B. G., Stueve, A., & Pescosolido, B. A. (2000). Public conceptions of mental illness in 1950 and 1996: What is mental illness and is it to be feared? *Journal of Health and Social Behavior, 41*, 188–207.
Pingani, L., Forghieri, M., Ferrari, S., Ben-Zeev, D., Artoni, P., Mazzi, F., et al. (2012). Stigma and discrimination toward mental illness: Translation and validation of the Italian version of the attribution questionnaire-27 (AQ-27-I). *Social Psychiatry and Psychiatric Epidemiology, 47*(6), 993–999.
Radcliffe, P., & Stevens, A. (2008). Are drug treatment services only for 'thieving junkie scumbags'? Drug users and the management of stigmatised identities. *Social Science & Medicine, 67*(7), 1065–1073.
Rivera, A. V., DeCuir, J., Crawford, N. D., Amesty, S., & Lewis, C. F. (2014). Internalized stigma and sterile syringe use among people who inject drugs in new York City, 2010–2012. *Drug and Alcohol Dependence, 144*, 259–264.

Ronzani, T. M., Furtado, E. F., & Higgins-Biddle, J. (2009). Stigmatization of alcohol and other drug users by primary care providers in Southeast Brazil. *Social Science & Medicine, 69*(7), 1080–1084.

Room, R., Rehm, J., Trotter, R. T., II, Paglia, A., & Üstün, T. B. (2001). Cross-cultural views on stigma valuation parity and societal attitudes towards disability. In T. B. Üstün, S. Chatterji, J. E. Bickenbach, R. T. Trotter II, R. Room, & J. Rehm (Eds.), *Disability and culture: Universalism and diversity* (pp. 247–291). Hofgrebe & Huber: Seattle, WA.

Schomerus, G., Lucht, M., Holzinger, A., Matschinger, H., Carta, M. G., & Angermeyer, M. C. (2011). The stigma of alcohol dependence compared with other mental disorders: A review of population studies. *Alcohol and Alcoholism, 46*(2), 105–112.

Silveira, P. S. S., Casela, A. L. M., Monteiro, É. P., Ferreira, G. C. L., Freitas, J. V., Machado, N. M., Noto, A. N., & Ronzani, T. M. (2016). Psychosocial understanding of self-stigma among people who seek treatment for drug addiction. *Stigma and Health, 22*, 1–16. https://doi.org/10.1037/sah0000069.

Silveira, P. S., Soares, R. G, Gomide, H. P., Ferreira, G. C.L., Casela, A. L. M., Martins, L. F., & Ronzani, T. M. (2015). Social distance toward people with substance dependence: A survey among health professionals. Psicologia em Pesquisa (UFJF), 9(2), 170–176.

Spencer, J., Deakin, J., Seddon, T., Ralphs, R., & Boyle, J. (2008). *Getting problem drug users (back) into employment.* London: UK Drug Policy Commission (UKDPC).

Ssebunnya, J., Kigozi, F., Lund, C., Kizza, D., & Okello, E. (2009). Stakeholder perceptions of mental health stigma and poverty in Uganda. *BMC International Health and Human Rights, 9*(1), 5.

Steele, C. M., & Aronson, J. (1995). Stereotype threat and the intellectual test performance of African Americans. *Journal of Personality and Social Psychology, 69*(5), 797.

van Boekel, L. C., Brouwers, E. P., van Weeghel, J., & Garretsen, H. F. (2013). Public opinion on imposing restrictions to people with an alcohol-or drug addiction: A cross-sectional survey. *Social Psychiatry and Psychiatric Epidemiology, 48*(12), 2007–2016.

van Olphen, J., Eliason, M. J., Freudenberg, N., & Barnes, M. (2009). Nowhere to go: How stigma limits the options of female drug users after release from jail. *Substance Abuse Treatment, Prevention, and Policy, 4*(1), 10.

Weiss, L., McCoy, K., Kluger, M., & Finkelstein, R. (2004). Access to and use of health care: Perceptions and experiences among people who use heroin and cocaine. *Addiction Research & Theory, 12*(2), 155–165.

West, M. L., Yanos, P. T., & Mulay, A. L. (2014). Triple stigma of forensic psychiatric patients: Mental illness, race, and criminal history. *International Journal of Forensic Mental Health, 13*(1), 75–90.

WHO. (2016). *Public health dimension of the world drug problem.* Report by the Secretariat—Executive Board, 140th session, Provisional agenda item 10.3, EB140/29. World Health Organization, Geneva. Retrieved from http://apps.who.int/gb/ebwha/pdf_files/EB140/B140_29-en.pdf

Chapter 3
Social Effects of Prohibitionism in the Americas and New Drug Policies

Marcelo Rossal

Abstract The prohibitionist complex is still powerful and multiform. Despite the evil it has been proved to unleash, avoiding it is a tough task. On the one hand, this article focuses on the persistence of prohibitionism in Uruguay and the violence (both statal and interpersonal) that it inflicts on the most vulnerable drug users. On the other hand, it discusses the historical reasons why Uruguay has to challenge the prohibitionist complex and describes the specific civilizing path that resulted from other efforts to modify drug policies. In Uruguay, alcohol and prostitution have historically been regulated and controlled by the State, with an approach that has privileged public health rather than moral considerations. By contrast, challenges to prohibitionism are more market-centered in the United States than in Uruguay. Prohibitionism is in decline in both cases, either by direct state action or by regulation through the production of a legal market and taxes.

3.1 Introduction

This chapter focuses on the social effects of prohibitionism and the ways that different societies, with different civilizing processes, have found to abandon such a paradigm.

First, I define prohibitionism as a transnational complex that assembles different beliefs, interest groups, legal instruments, and institutions that fight for the elimination of any use of drugs that they define as illegal according to criteria defined over time, but inevitably rooted in the ethnocentric conceptions of early twentieth-century progressivism (Courtwright 2014).

Second, based on ethnographic experience, I focus on the drug policy of Uruguay, which is a country marked by a civilizing process that has made the State the guarantor and protector of the individual in different dimensions, especially regarding health. More progressive than liberal, the Uruguayan state has taken over the regula-

M. Rossal (✉)
Universidad de la República, Montevideo, Uruguay
e-mail: mrossal@fhuce.edu.uy

T. M. Ronzani (ed.), *Drugs and Social Context*,
https://doi.org/10.1007/978-3-319-72446-1_3

tion of cannabis with the idea of protecting the health and safety of citizens. Analyzing the case, it is notorious that the country has preserved, and even radicalized, elements of the "War on Drugs" and that the greatest efforts have been directed to fighting against cocaine base paste supply. Meanwhile, the cannabis market has been regulated through bold legislation that has defied the international drug control regime and the very core of the prohibitionist complex.

Third, I compare the Uruguayan case to the American case. In the USA, the civilizing process is liberal and mostly Protestant. The prohibitionist complex is rooted in the protection of individual freedom that characterizes some states, and it has been interwoven with criticism about the high costs of the War on Drugs (Brumm and Cloninger 1994; Friedman 1991). Thus, in some states, formulae that protect the individual rights of consumers and provide them with regulated market access to cannabis flourish. According to well-reputed neoclassical economists, this is the best way to regulate substances (Becker et al. 2004). Oscillating between puritanical prohibition and liberal regulation through the market, the US federal government keeps a prohibitionist system of international control over the rest of the world. Meanwhile, in many of its states, citizens defend their liberties through referendums and the federal government can do little to prevent them. (Thoumi 2013). Eventually, as the drug normalization process continues to grow (Martínez Oró 2015), it is possible to visualize a large part of the US population making use of cannabis legal (Graham 2015).

3.2 Moralism, Hygienism, and Drug Policies

Alcohol and other drug policies have been marked by a century of controversy. I do not intend to dwell on this history, but instead to focus on an issue that has been the moral and ideological basis of drug policies since the late nineteenth century: improvement of the human species from different perspectives. One of the historical bases of prohibitionism had its origins in the leagues that had fought since the nineteenth century, mainly in the USA, against the consumption of alcohol and against other "social vices," including prostitution. These groups added a moral and religious dimension to the evidence that supported the advance of hygienism (Levine and Reinarman 1991). At that time, the USA and Uruguay devised different solutions to the same problem. While Uruguay tried to regulate health risks from an active State initiative, in the USA the debate was between prohibition and freedom. Uruguay regulated prostitution and the production of alcohol, whereas in the USA the Puritan solution prevailed, first in communities where the party supporting prohibitionism had greater influence, and then in the whole country. In Uruguay, there is still a consensus regarding the need to defend public health from threats of risky consumption, and the current solution is still based on regulation with a strong presence of the State.

From the moral point of view, prohibitionist policies defend a free human against alienation. This modern ambition, which combines with an opposition to ideological conceptions (although being quite paradoxical), has served to protect actual women and men but also to reduce their spaces of freedom and push them to maximum alienation when taking any decision. Until the 1980s, within both capitalism and Soviet communism, it was agreed that it was necessary to ban certain substances that were not prescribed by doctors. This showed a world that was bipolar in many aspects, but absolutely hegemonic in the model of mental health imposed on the inhabitants of the planet (Wiseman 1985). This unipolarity of the hegemonic medical model was challenged from within the medical field as well as from the outside. The countercultural revolution initiated in the 1960s in the West called the model into question, especially regarding what was referred to as drug use. This countercultural revolution resulted in a number of new rights regarding both individuals and ethnic communities.

Also in the 1960s, in parallel to the countercultural revolution taking place, theoretical perspectives were being broadened. The focus of the reflections about contemporary societies shifted to social class; moreover, ethnic-racial and gender issues were incorporated in order to understand and face inequalities.

Nineteenth-century eugenics sought strong healthy workers within racially and ideologically pure national spaces. After World War II, the defeat of Nazi fascism, the massive access to the world of work by women, and the process of decolonization created the conditions for a global expansion in the rights of individuals and put a brake on certain ambitions for "improvement" of the species. Nonetheless, the United Nations (UN), the instrument for strengthening human rights around the world, quickly became polarized and plagued by regional conflicts. The UN also became the arena for discussions on how to expand and guarantee rights while controlling planetary security by having weapons capable of mass extermination. The countries with the greatest extermination capacity established themselves as permanent members of the UN Security Council and began to arbitrate in different conflicts. The board had two heads, the USA and the Soviet Union. On the positive side, the USA could represent the ambition of universal individual liberty while the Soviet Union could account for the ambition of real equality. The universalist revolutionary triad of liberty, equality, and fraternity, with different emphases, was well represented and had won the war against Nazi particularism. With certain fraternity, the different peoples of the world could aspire to configure humanity.

The development of the Cold War is a story with a known end: For the sake of a realpolitik charged with particular interests, the USA supported regimes such as Latin American dictatorships that flagrantly violated freedom. Meanwhile, the Soviet Union also did so, corrupting regimes that were based on the most violent inequality. Through five decades, the so-called Cold War prompted extremely bloody wars, missile crises, revolutions, and attacks of all kinds. However, in some cases consensus was achieved. It was often produced by the field work of transnational agencies, which had their own economic resources and agendas that did not affect the issues of controversy between the superpowers. The prohibition of drug use and exchange was one of the exceptions and it stretched over the pre- and post-Cold War periods. Such measures were the fruit of the association of breeder selectors and moral entrepreneurs, who disseminated a drug biopolitics propaganda based on two fundamental pillars: the hegemonic medical model (Menéndez 1985) and Puritan morality (Morone 1997), which had its communist correlate in the search for the "new man" (Wiseman 1985). For such types of moral subjectivity, drugs are not admissible (i.e., those drugs not allowed by their respective cultures).

Regarding the Uruguayan case, the Cold War influenced shaping of the "drug problem" through the creation of a specialized police unit, at a time when the authorities of the Uruguayan dictatorship supported by the USA did not consider the *drugs* as a relevant issue. In the context of Nixon's push for the War on Drugs, US officials encouraged the creation of a Uruguayan antinarcotics police unit based on the intelligence department. Even though the 1974 Uruguayan legislation had not criminalized the use of any of the substances prohibited by the international antidrug system, the victims of that police unit started to appear shortly after (Castro 2015).

In any case, the USA had already benefited from a fertile ground associating the puritanism momentarily in office with the (bio)politicians of the early twentieth century, and bringing such conjunction to a radical extreme in the concept of a "Dry Country." The prohibition of alcohol only lasted the brief period it did because it quickly damaged the health of problematic users and the good manners that it wanted to protect, but also because it favored an exponential growth of organized crime. Moreover, it was a failed policy because it affronted the beliefs of several ethnic Caucasian groups that lived in the USA and had been gaining significant political and social power (Musto 1999). Regarding other drugs, the prohibitions could be maintained because offenses were legitimized by racism. The prohibitions remained untouched because racism itself was one of the foundations (Lusane and Desmond 1991).

Likewise, the prohibition of drug use affected mainly those subjects who had previously been unequally treated and structurally displaced: the poor, the non-whites and, during some years, the women. Throughout the Americas, prisons are filled with drug traffickers, which shows how effective prohibitionism is in generating both state violence and violence within society. It triggers both internal violence within the illicit market and symbolic violence against drug users. In some social contexts, in addition to stigmatization, drug users receive the punishment of criminalization and the violent responses that are systemic to the illicit market.

Prohibitionism punishes differently according to the country, but in the most precarious circuits of the illegal market, lives of the poorest of all nations turn equal. For most of the subjects involved in the traffic circuits, prohibitionism produces as much violence as precarious economic opulence. The circulation of money and certain objects of consumption do not guarantee improvement in the lives of the poor, but there is an exponential increase in violence in their communities and in their relations with more violent and, in some cases, more corrupt states (Auyero et al. 2014).

In geopolitical terms, there are some differences between the diverse impacts of prohibitionism. In the richest countries, most of the drug-related deaths are due to overdoses and problems derived from illicit drug consumption. Meanwhile, in Latin American countries, the inverse is true, with violent deaths being much more systemically related to the illegal market than those caused by the use of drugs. This does not mean that there is no state violence towards users or systemic violence among traffickers in in rich countries, the key point is that state sovereignty is more precarious in weaker states, impunity is greater, and state violence is bloodier. The wars against drugs initiated in the 1980s made first Colombia and then Mexico, as well as other countries and regions of other Latin American nations, the scenarios of incremental state violence. Because an increase in state violence usually corrupts officials and corrodes institutions, violence and impunity go hand in hand.

I could see in the field that the higher the radicalization of state violence against drugs, the more disastrous the results are. Both negative consequences increase; the production of criminal violence increases and the social suffering of illicit substance users also deepens. A policy that was established to protect public health has ended up increasing pain and worsening the indicators of criminology.

Focusing on the case of users of cocaine paste base can help in understanding these sufferings as well as the worsening of data related to criminal violence. In Uruguay, a country that has undertaken a historic change in the way of dealing with drug policy, we can see the complex courses of action that prohibitionism takes in the multiform framework of its decline. Relating the persistent prohibitionist approach to the use of cocaine paste base and the almost opposite approach to the use of cannabis offers us a "live" laboratory of the drug policies that are currently being implemented.

3.3 Drug Policies in Uruguay

The Uruguayan case is interesting because it is a Latin American country that is not characterized by extreme poverty, extreme criminal violence, or having a weak state. However, certain sectors of the metropolitan area of Montevideo that are endemically affected by abject poverty experienced a significant increase in population between the 1990s and the crisis of 2002. These areas thus became the scenarios of cocaine base paste consumption and marketing, and of the systemic violence associated with trafficking of the substance.

The market for illicit drugs in Uruguay is notoriously fragmented regarding the drugs and their different uses. Cocaine base paste and synthetic drugs are substances consumed by people with very different trajectories; they do not come across each other, either spatially or socially, and even participate in completely detached markets. In the middle- and upper-class neighborhoods of Montevideo there are synthetic drugs users, but users of cocaine base paste are almost non-existent. By contrast, in the lower-class neighborhoods of the city, there are not many synthetic drugs users but many more cocaine base users. Synthetic drugs are associated with users who enjoy a kind of extended youth and recreation in electronic parties; they are people with university degrees and participation in the labor market. The substances come from Europe through networks that link the users without generating major conflicts. In the drug use care records, the contact is usually listed because of some isolated intoxication. (Rossal and Suárez 2016).

In contrast, cocaine paste is carried in trucks from the Andean heart of South America. Its users, in general, have been consuming the substance for many years and often do not have the capacity to pay for it. Every day, they experience conflictive situations with the police, the traffickers, and their neighbors. They are the most stigmatized subjects of the working class neighborhoods and usually cannot keep their jobs, which are certainly informal or even part of the illegal market. These are people who have had less than 7 years of formal schooling (60%), who have lived on the streets and in shelters (30%), and have had contact with the penal system (50%) (Suárez and Ramírez 2014). Many cocaine base paste users have undergone a treatment process, which often complies with forms of institutional violence such as the asylum or therapeutic community models that involve physical confrontation, punishment, and experiencing the "therapeutic" action of stigma. The average age of the cocaine paste base user population has increased, which suggests that there are few new users and that this market has stopped growing (Suárez and Ramírez 2014).

The exchange of cocaine base paste occurs in a context of extreme violence, in which users of the substance, traffickers, prisons, agents of the penal system, legislation, political speeches, and journalism are assembled. The stigmatizing discourses find an agent in the punitive inflation and end up punishing drug users. Through my research, I have been able to appreciate firsthand the corporeal and emotional punishment that everyday cocaine paste base users suffer and how this sanction is directly related to prohibitionism and the application of a punitive approach to reducing the supply of drugs.

Uruguay's drug policies have been understood as liberal and have been characterized as progressive.[1] But, a quick reading could lead to misunderstandings. Uruguay has been marked by an active State with an early social protection system, in which public health and the power of physicians was central (Barrán 1992).

Since the end of the nineteenth century, in addition to an increasing medical coverage, primary, secular, free, and compulsory education defined a kind of practical civil religion (Guigou 2003). It succeeded in producing a secular sense of social life within majoritarian sectors and conceiving a series of terrestrial rights to be guaranteed by the State, relegating religiosity to the private world and to intimacy (Caetano 2011).

In such a way, the Uruguayan state assumed massive social, sanitary, and educational tasks with almost missionary aims. The *Batllista* proposal of the State as a "shield of the weak" flourished in many different welfare areas and outlined what Milton Vagner (Vanger 1983) later called the "model country." Uruguay, the best consolidated democracy in South America, had its foundation in secularism and social protection, as well as in the centrality of the power of medical doctors. Moreover, for a short period during the 1930s, abortion was allowed in the country. Although such legislation was enacted during a dictatorship, it was voted in by a parliament that had debated different visions of the issue; the eugenic and hygienist arguments had exceeded the religious ones, at least among the representatives of the dominant classes (Sapriza 2002).

Since the first decade of the twentieth century, a State entity had been projected to take charge of policies related to oil and alcohol (Martínez 2010). It sought to

---

[1] http://latitude.blogs.nytimes.com/2013/08/21/cannabis-country/, http://www.nytimes.com/2013/08/01/world/americas/uruguay-lawmakers-to-vote-on-legalizing-marijuana.html

safeguard the country from the international oil trust and to protect the health of the population by producing alcohols as a monopoly. By doing so, the Uruguayan state regulated alcohol; meanwhile, the USA banned it. Faced with the same problem ("alcoholism"), the Uruguayan solution was far from punitive; it was based on a regulationist State.[2] The same had already been done with prostitution. In contrast to the extended Puritan prohibitionism and Anglo-Saxon liberalism, Uruguayan solutions were geared toward state protection.

The way that the young people who defend the individual right to smoke cannabis misunderstand the figure of José Mujica explains it clearly:

> Marijuana consumers around the world hailed him. His face appears on T-shirts and paraphernalia with the iconic leaf and Rastafarian colors. But he says that the young people who congratulate him do not understand his intention: "Smoke-free, bullshit! It has nothing to do with freedom; for me, it is a security problem, it is against drug trafficking. I have rotted to explain it. But people want to hear what they think "(Müller and Draper 2017, p. 275).

Lawyers Diego Silva Forné (2016) and Pablo Galaín (2015) clearly explain that Law No. 19.172 on the regulation and control of cannabis is based on a model of user health protection (i.e., harm reduction), which was assumed by Uruguay during the first decade of the century. Beyond protecting the freedom of users to consume the substance, the ideas that underlie the Uruguayan legislation are rooted in the protection of health and public security as a challenge against illegal drug traffic.

During the twentieth century, Uruguay adhered to the different prohibitionist conventions, but despite the escalation of prohibitions on the use of certain substances (cannabis, coca leaf derivatives, and opium derivatives), the country maintained its profile: drug use is a matter of population health, and the use of drugs has not been explicitly criminalized since the 1970s. However, the forms of health protection of those times were highly tutelary and, of course, some forms of health care can (literally) imply various violations against fundamental rights.

[2] In the 1990s, during a neoliberal momentum in the region, the state monopoly on alcohol was repealed. During the parliamentary debate, progressivism defended the state monopoly of alcohol by arguing health protection. Senator Astori (current Minister of Economy and the main political orchestrator of the "progressive era" economic policy) pointed out at a Senate session on 24 October 1995, "It seems to us that what is at stake is a public or collective good. One of these the market cannot supply, so they must be generated by other means. I hold that control of an important part of public health is at stake, and this is a public good that the market does not ensure. I am going to support a good part of my argument on that subject, just as I did in the Constitution and Legislation Commission". http://www.parlamento.gub.uy/sesiones/AccesoSesiones.asp?Url=/sesiones/diarios/senado/html/19951024s0056.htm

3.4 Between Harm Reduction, the Criminal System, and the Tutelary Disposition of the Progressive State

In 2004, Uruguayan drug policies officially assumed the reduction of risks and damages as a transversal policy for all state sectors, including those relating to sanitary, legal, or social protection. Based on such policy, the State began to call for proposals for social projects to deal with drug use and the new cannabis legislation.

However, beyond the official drug policy, practice is much more complex. A relational scenario was drawn by two oppositions: prohibitionism/decriminalization and abstention/reduction of damages. Although the dominant correspondence usually assimilates prohibitionism with abstention and decriminalization with damage reduction (Loeck 2014), the existence of "hygienist" models of harm reduction can also be seen in the ethnographic field, along with extreme abstentionism that supports decriminalization. Thus, these two oppositions, instead of narrowing the relational scenario, allow for a series of combinations and a complex and open classification that is difficult to define accurately. Moreover, the arena became more complex when associations of users or their relatives and families entered the scene.[3]

The emergence of user organizations had a clear public impact. In the case of cannabis users, they could fully tension the postulates of the official policies. Following Bourdieu (1997), these cannabis users were possessors of significant social, cultural, and even economic capitals; therefore, they could concur the agency of their efforts together with that of several national and international actors and achieve the approval of a law that protected them in their use of the substance. They attained such a goal despite adverse public opinion polls, divided medical opinions, and internal dissent within the governing party (Müller and Draper 2017). Certainly, some organized cannabis users and growers were able to place themselves at the center of the scene (i.e., in power) and they generated new demands to their left and new displacements toward the right. For instance, one the one hand, some users have refused to register themselves as growers; on the other hand, the detractors of the new law have been marginalized and considered part of the "conservative Uruguay," as had happened with those who opposed other progressive laws of Mujica's government (Arocena and Aguiar 2017). However, the new legislation protects all cannabis users and growers because, with certain restrictions, it detaches them from the criminal scope.

---

[3] Cannabis users' organizations have been advocates of total decriminalization and harm reduction for the use of all substances, but associations of family members of users of cocaine base (the first that took public voice was significantly called "Mothers of the square") have held a position of desperate extreme abstentionism, with an understandably tutelary but not criminalizing imprint. The Facebook page of "Madres de la Plaza" proposed on 26 November 2014: "Compulsive hospitalization of addicts in public and private centers under the care of qualified staff, under the close supervision of mothers and relatives; eradicate from the streets all those who, victims of this terrible disease, have become a danger to themselves, their families and for the whole of society; we propose the creation of treatment centers, therapeutic communities, farms, and special spaces intended for the rehabilitation and physical and mental recovery of the sick."

As a counterpoise to organized cannabis users, cocaine base users are stigmatized; they have a negative symbolic capital. They lack any power and the legislation in force, especially that approved in the last period of government, does not establish protective measures but increases the punitive pressure over them.

3.5 Contradictions in Uruguayan Drug Policy? Other Scenarios for the War on Drugs?

Contradictions would be a mark of the country's drug policy if such duality – protection of socially integrated sectors and daily punishment of the poorest – was not a long-term trend in the country.

Let us examine this question in more detail. Concurrent with the cannabis regulation law, which was more protective and state-centric than liberal, increased penalties were imposed on trafficking cocaine base paste compared with trafficking of other illegal drugs under Law No. 19,007. According to the prosecutor Carlos Negro (2013), it is a "bad law": "[...] not only because of the technical defects in its formulation but also because of its purposes, public policy for tackling a health problem such as abuse of illegal drugs." Another jurist, Gianella Bardazano (2014) explicitly points out the contradiction of drug policies in Uruguay. However, this issue could be seen from a different perspective: the Uruguayan state follows a tutelary tradition in relation to its citizens, especially in what is referred to as public space, no matter the approach from which we understand the term "public space." Although Law 19,007 increases the penal pressure on users of cocaine paste base because they are inevitably involved in the network of exchanges of the substance, Faults Law No. 19,120 affected them to a greater extent (based on our ethnographic experience). This is the legal instrument that allows daily police punishment to the *pastosos*,[4] following an old tradition of punishment to the unfit poor.

Police violence increased in the USA as the effect of aggressive policing forms derived from the broken windows theory (Wacquant, 2010, 2012). In Uruguay, the Law of Faults increased the practical powers of police officers to coerce cocaine base paste users who spend every night on the streets and squares. Decriminalizing drug use does not guarantee that users will not be punished through the discretionary power of judges to apply legal forms such as "non-consumption tenure." The case of decriminalization of drug use in Portugal was successful because it had a robust policy oriented toward the care of drug users (Hughes and Stevens 2010). By contrast, in Uruguay, where consumption has already been decriminalized, harm reduction is more theory than consistent practice, because legal access to a drug is not yet guaranteed for the most vulnerable populations. Currently, the risks and damages to users need to be guaranteed, not regarding the health consequences of substance use, but the possibility of being criminally punished and suffering the deleterious effects of imprisonment or psychiatric confinement.

---

[4] Pejorative term used to refer to cocaine paste users who stroll through streets, squares, and parks or spend the night sleeping rough.

3.6 Effects of Prohibition on Users of Cocaine Base Paste

As we have seen, according to the available data (Suárez and Ramírez 2014), almost 50% of the Uruguayan problematic users of cocaine paste base, both adults and adolescents, have been affected by the penal system a third of them live on the streets or in shelters for the homeless, which also implies subjection to the same stigma as living on the street (Panter-Brick 2002).

As shown in previous research on the trajectories of the inhabitants of the street, institutional violence is the dimension that consolidates such stigma (Fraiman and Rossal 2011). In other words, violence occurs not only during passage through the prison system, but also child protection institutions, daily police detentions (even if no crime has been committed), and stays in shelters. The institutional procedures of these places serve to consolidate (and introject) the stigma, which for the Uruguayan case are emblematized by the term *pichi*. This degrading term is used by many police officers as a synonym for delinquent and, in slang, as a synonym for vulnerable person.

In times of the "model country," torture was a police practice dedicated to *pichis* (Albano et al. 2015). As a counterpoise to its civilization process (Elias 1988), the Uruguayan state continues to punish its poorest citizens, for whom it allocates focused social protection instruments that function through "advanced liberal" forms of governmentality (Rose et al. 2012), which are marked by the precariousness of their technicians.[5]

Thus, from this mode of governmentality, social policy devices oriented toward the achievement of central civilizing objectives such as harm reduction, gender equality, and violence prevention have been developed "on the territory." Using international or budgetary funds (depending on the case), the left hand of the State (Bourdieu 1999) operates in the protection of sectors targeted by their risk and vulnerability: women with children affected by domestic violence; young people who do not study or work; and drug users. These programs deplete their economic resources in the short terms of their contracts; thus, they hire technicians for short periods. Meanwhile, the repressive and tutelary facets of the State operate through immovable civil servants.

To face state punishment (whether legal or not), the State, this complex multiplicity, offers the most vulnerable people the attention of technicians who also work in precarious conditions. The country's policies, which are usually underlined as part of a long-term "civilizing" and "progressive" scheme, remain in the long-term line of punishing the *pichis*.

---

[5] In Latin America, "neoliberal governmentality" has a negative meaning and it sound offensive to the experts: social technicians, educators, and volunteers from these forms of governmentality that Nikolas Rose characterizes as advanced liberal. Certainly, these focused types of attention to the most precarious subjects through short-term projects that also turn social work precarious are characteristic of neoliberal policies. Wacquant (2012, p 508) points out: "The terms 'postsocial governance,' 'advanced liberal,' and 'late liberal' are often used as synonyms for neoliberal."

In particular, the Law of Faults constituted a systematic increase in state violence against the users of cocaine paste base and a re-legitimation of the daily police action toward the *pastosos*, epitome of the *pichis*. To get an idea of this everyday punitive pressure, some data are very eloquent: There are approximately 1150 available beds in homeless shelters belonging to the Ministry of Social Development, a large number of their users being cocaine base consumers. Out of a total of no more than 10,000 users of cocaine base in Montevideo, more than the 30% have had periods of sleeping rough on the streets and are precisely the cocaine paste base users who undergo the greatest difficulties. In addition, within the first 70 days of its enforcement, the Law of Faults prompted 1036 police interventions and 127 detentions. No prosecutions occurred, because the law states the need for a minimum of two interventions for the judge to be able to dictate a sentence.[6] These figures give a clear idea of the daily pressure and institutional violence this population suffers.

As described elsewhere (Fraiman and Rossal 2011), institutional violence consolidates stigma by the passage through tutelary spaces that mark the trajectories of the subjects; prisons and asylums for adolescents are spaces of citizenship loss. In this sense, institutional violence is the equivalent of political violence in the violence continuum scheme proposed by Bourgois (2009). The author shows four forms of violence that form a continuum: structural violence, symbolic violence, normalized violence, and political violence.

Although the brutalities are naturalized (naturalized violence) in tutelary spaces, the stigmas are internalized (symbolic violence) and the majority of violence ensures the reproduction of criminalization among those who use cocaine base. Likewise, the laws are responsible for the perpetuation of punishment of the poor; As Bourgois (2009, p. 30) recalls, quoting Benjamin, "for the marginalized, every day is a state of emergency."

However, these are not the only situations that cause criminal justice to be imparted to the users of cocaine paste. One of my interlocutors (Alejo, 30 years old) went to jail in the midst of a deranged maelstrom that had him as protagonist: After consuming for 3 days, he took a bicycle from a garden and fell asleep by its side. He was awakened by a police officer, bullied, and then prosecuted and imprisoned. Another user of cocaine base (Agustín, 26 years old) borrowed a cell phone from a casual street acquaintance and left his backpack behind with his identity card inside. Soon after, he lost the phone and all contact with the guy. Some months later, he was asked for his identification on the street and when giving his name, it came up that he was a wanted offender. The result was the same: prosecution and imprisonment. State violence begins as bureaucratic violence. In both cases, imprisonment was imposed on subjects that need, unequivocally, to be protected in their rights to health care. However, the State sent them to the lowest ranked place in prison classification: the "addict prisoner," the "*rake* (insignificant thief) without codes," the "dirty" without family or assistance of any kind.[7]

[6] http://www.elpais.com.uy/informacion/indigentes-dia-son-detenidos-policia.html

[7] During interviews with people imprisoned before 2002, the arrival of new prisoners, generally *rakes*, emerges as a topic. In general, the *rakes* are prosecuted by causes of trifle, thefts of small

By imparting justice to its most vulnerable subjects in this way, the Uruguayan state is feeding violence rather than stopping it, mainly in those areas of urban territory most subject to the dynamics of the illegal market. In recent years, during a process of radicalization of urban segregation, homicides have increased because of an increase in "systemic" interpersonal violence (Goldstein 1985; Reuter 2009) within the cocaine base market.[8] Violence in robberies has also increased in the poorest neighborhoods of Montevideo and its metropolitan area. A report that covers the first semester of 2015, shows that the regions of Montevideo inhabited by the middle and upper classes have "European" homicide rates (less than 2/100,000 inhabitants); meanwhile, in the poorest neighborhoods, homicide rates reached the same figures as in Mexico (more than 20/100,000 inhabitants).[9]

During the years that I have been carrying out research on the use of cocaine base, I have not stopped seeing bullet and knife wounds that dozens of my interlocutors have shown me. They showed me their wounds, but very few told me the reasons for the aggression, nor did they tell the judicial agents. One interlocutor told me that he had been injured by the son of his former partner, but because he did not report him they finally made up. During the last 2 years, I have interviewed two users of the health system who entered the hospital with gunshot wounds. Being kind and collaborative, these men narrated their life trajectories to me reflexively and exhaustively, but they were evasive about the injuries that took them to the hospital. The continuity of violence also serves to reproduce impunity and the spirals of aggression and distrust.

3.7 Guardianship

The word "tutelar" is not appreciated in the field of human rights protection. For instance, policies existing before the adoption of the new Codes of Childhood and Adolescence are characterized as tutelary, but indigenous reservations and hospices are also tutelary. In the case of children and the family, tutelary care has been

---

amounts related to the urgent need to obtain resources for use of cocaine base paste. There are also cases of cell phone thefts from pedestrians, sometimes threatened with small knives. Although this is a crime that has a penalty that imposes imprisonment, within the prison population those who make these small assaults are not considered professional thieves, but *rakes*. In a previous work, through an ethnographic scene we can see how a prisoner self-considered a criminal treats the other subject he considers just a "dirty."

[8] Technicians and authorities from the Ministry of Interior explained that the increase in the number of homicides, which soared in 2012, was due to "settlements" among people with criminal records, many of them linked to the market of illicit substances. In 2012, homicides increased by 34% compared to 2011. https://www.minterior.gub.uy/observatorio/images/stories/datos2012.pdf

[9] http://www.elobservador.com.uy/barrios-montevideo-tasa-homicidios-similar-mexico-n671953 It is shocking to appreciate the rapid increase in violence in some regions of Mexico in parallel with the repressive push of the War on Drugs and the impunity and corruption of state institutions (Azaola 2012).

opposed to protection, which has been complemented by another term to become "integral protection." Moreover, tutelary care has become a paradigmatic issue and a kind of hegemonic preaching in academic fields in international organizations. But, it has not yet become dominant among Uruguayan political leaders.

Former President Mujica has more than once pointed out the need to relocate cocaine paste users to the countryside, and such a response has even been requested by relatives of some of these users.[10] Some treatment plans do actually work by relocating users to isolated areas. Others impose corporeal punishment and force their inmates to adhere to religious beliefs that they often do not share. Some others, headed by university professionals,[11] charge large sums of money to the users' families. One can identify these devices in the speech of the interlocutors because there is always only one way of leaving: escape.

These hospices located in the countryside are healthy and hygienic places, but patients' rights are suspended so that they can be later reintegrated into society. They represent a currently unacceptable solution, but remain at the core of many Uruguayans beliefs. This tutelary system is supported by people from different social backgrounds, from the right and left, from civil servants and labor union advocates to practitioners of the Pentecostal faith.[12]

An interlocutor I came across in the field was an intelligent and wise 75-year-old lady, who was the grandmother of a young cocaine base paste user who had lived on the streets for some years. She described hopefully, but at the same time with doubt, her project to get users off the streets and relocate them into a community or colony in the countryside. Her plan involved several state institutions and ministries responsible for public security, social protection, public health, and education. Her project contained a well-thought-out organization chart, which included the university and scientific research.

---

[10] At the beginning of his presidential term, José Mujica, the president who enacted the laws of equal marriage, cannabis regulation, and abortion, proposed that cocaine base paste users would use military service or rural activities as a way to "get them out of their places and put them to do physical work" http://www.infobae.com/2010/03/26/507854-jose-mujica-propone-un-servicio-militar-los-adictos-al-paco

[11] One of these therapeutic communities uses as therapy the total separation of adolescent drug users from their entire family for 3 months, the aim being to detoxify him/her and modify their relational familiar patterns. In an interview with a user's grandmother, the interviewee pointed out to some family member that she had not complied with the treatment because she had celebrated the adolescent's birthday, before that period. The teen eventually escaped from the place, which, of course, is a result of confinement that deprives a teenager of seeing their family for 3 months.

[12] Faced with the proposed closure of psychiatric "colonies," the public health workers' union defended the continuity of these colonies, living museums of tutelary times in which locked-up citizens suffered all kinds of violence. In 2006, the new progressive government intended to close these colonies for a couple of years, a proposal the union opposed. In 2016, almost a decade later, the government has still not closed the colonies despite denouncing them. Today, as in 2006, the union opposes closure. On the other hand, two organizations of Pentecostal origin have communities in rural areas in which they deal with the "rehabilitation of addicts" by separation from their places of origin. http://www.espectador.com/sociedad/59632/msp-pretende-cerrar-las-colonias-psiquiatricas-etchepare-y-santin-carlos-rossi y http://ladiaria.com.uy/articulo/2015/8/en-transito/

When I was asked about my opinion on the project, I answered with another question: "Do you know the state psychiatric colonies?" She answered by recounting the names of colonies, even mentioning some I had never heard about, such as the Hansen Institute where lepers and other patients with incurable diseases were hospitalized. A relative of hers had lived there in the 1950s. She recounted the events with horror and described those perverse spaces of decitizenization, where people were abandoned to the darkest spaces of the State, even though this had been the most opulent moment of the Uruguayan state in its whole history. In the conversation, we fearfully remembered that, in one of the state psychiatric colonies, a pack of dogs had recently killed an intern, and that a number of irregularities were brought to light after that 2015 case.[13]

3.8 Normalization and Civilizing Processes

Gregor Burkhart, a well-known expert at the European Monitoring Center for Drugs and Drug Addiction, referred to a civilizing process when characterizing the policies that prevent the use of harmful substances and compares them with other civilizational limitations of social life: "The strategies that limit or de-popularize tobacco consumption and excessive use of alcohol follow this evolution of 'civilizing' public life (just like traffic lights and the prohibition of spitting on the ground) and at the same time try to sort out market policy failures" (Burkhart 2009, p. 392). In the conclusions of his article, the European Union expert recommends policies combining drug use restrictions in coordination with harm reduction, adding: "On the other hand, it is conceptually and historically incorrect to seek similarities with Prohibition of the 1930s in the USA or with fascism because when environmental strategies put restrictions on behavior, they are just limited to the sphere of public life" (Burkhart 2009, p. 393).

It is necessary to recognize that the approach is interesting: policies that restrict certain practices are not fascist because they regulate the behaviors that produce collective life, such as respecting traffic lights. However, drug regulations that specifically ban substances should be considered differently. These substances are authorized by the existence of civilizing processes that have allowed the development of individuals within societies that restrict the practices that violate their rights and bring down any form of violence. Thus, some restrictions on drugs use are legitimately exercised, whereas others may have a totalitarian character, such as penalizing the use of drugs in circumstances that do not harm any person apart from the consumer. Accordingly, the court of appeal in the Argentine Republic declared that the law that criminalizes the cultivation of cannabis is unconstitutional.[14]

---

[13] http://www.elpais.com.uy/informacion/murio-paciente-mordido-perros-etchepare.html

[14] http://www.lanacion.com.ar/1531397-la-justicia-declara-inconstitucional-castigar-el-cultivo-de-marihuana-para-consumo-personal

Uruguayan Law No. 19.172 was conceived in light of the same civilizing sense. It deals with regulation of the whole cycles of distribution and use of cannabis (with the same restrictions as tobacco smoking, regarding smoked use of the substance; and the same restrictions as alcohol, concerning the driving of vehicles and machinery). In Uruguay, as already pointed out, drug use is decriminalized so such civilizing solutions should develop in the direction proposed by Burkhart, regulating the uses that could harm third parties or the public sphere. But, to arrive at this civilizing moment, some European and American countries still need to go through the decriminalization of the uses of drugs; in fact, they must remove the use of psychoactive substances from the criminal sphere.

Therefore, Western Europe and the Americas are the two main arenas of the debate on how to deal with the adverse effects of the War on Drugs, which has been sustained on a global scale for decades. In both locations, qualitative changes in the nature of civilization are taking place. The recent 2016 United Nations General Assembly Special Session on Drugs (UNGASS) made it possible to share the global state of the art with transparency, although its main features had already been discussed in the European context and in the Organization of American States (OAS) meeting of 2012. The second decade of the twenty-first century is seeing the breakdown of the War-on-Drugs hegemony, and how the slogan of "a world free of drugs" is dystopian. Accordingly, 2016 UNGASS has adopted a more realistic view that advocates "a world free of drug abuse."

In Latin America, the consequences of the crusade under the motto "a drug-free world" have resulted in a decline in the power of some nation-states to control sectors of their territories. This has been accompanied by an undeniable increase in corruption and hundreds of thousands of people killed and imprisoned. All these deprivations were suffered without obtaining the desired result. Instead, the opposite occurred: increased consumption of drugs and the growth, enrichment, and diversification of the illicit markets.

Considering such results, and that prevention campaigns based on shocking signs and slogans but dubious arguments have had iatrogenic effects for the direct users of the substances (Burkhart 2009), there is an urgent need for more sincere messages. The need for sincerity as the basic building block from which a new consensus can be reached seems to be a sign of the times.

For instance, the processes of cannabis use normalization and the perception of the use of marijuana as low risk go hand in hand; they are part of the same phenomenon for users and nonusers. People from the same generation usually consider that the use of cannabis is not so dangerous, due to their personal experience. In other words, users and their close friends know that cannabis does not have the risks attributed to it by prevention campaigns and prohibitionist speeches and that the use of cannabis carries no greater risk than that of tobacco or alcohol.

As I pointed out, The US case illustrates this process of normalization, with Barack Obama being eloquent on the subject: "Marijuana is no more dangerous than alcohol or tobacco."[15] Against this backdrop, cannabis use is authorized in different

[15] http://sociedad.elpais.com/sociedad/2014/01/19/actualidad/1390156784_083798.html

states, and different forms of market development for legal access to the substance are pragmatically provided.

Whether through state-centralized or market-centralized models,[16] the departure from prohibitionism is in the civilizing horizon of the West. This is in contrast to the situation in the Philippines, where an avowed admirer of Hitler's methods is leading a new dirty war against drug users.[17]

3.9 Conclusion

"Like the soldier who returns from the war and says we must stop" is how the supreme authority of the Uruguayan police feels (Müller and Draper 2017, p. 279). Uruguay has not been massively affected by the social and political effects of prohibitionism. However, different aspects of the global War on Drugs can be found in the poorest sectors of the metropolitan area of Montevideo and in some cities in the interior of the country. With the expansion of the drug market, many poor people live in permanent insecurity, and the war strategy has given no other result than increases in violence, imprisonment, corruption of institutions, and marginalization.

Throughout this paper, I have shown that there is no contradiction, but rather complementarity, in the Uruguayan policies aimed at people who use drugs: protection of socially integrated subjects and mistrust and punishment of the marginalized. The Uruguayan state maintains its protective imprint, reproducing it in its devices, agents, and many of its citizens. Those who do not know how to be a good citizen of the polis receive a tutelary response, state violence from the police, and are subjected to guardianship. However, even such common sense can break down. The defeat of prohibitionism regarding cannabis suggests a clear civilizing sense. We already know, thanks to the harm reduction policies of some parts of Europe, that facilitating legal access to different substances reduces state and social violence. Likewise, we know that policies should be aimed at combating violence, not feeding it.

At the margins of the Uruguayan state (Das and Poole 2004), the police and some parastate forms of social protection are governmental forms of advanced liberalism that operate in the targeting of marginalized subjects. The increase in state violence associated with repression of the most vulnerable correlates with the growth in violence within the illicit market to which they are subjected. Many of the people who use smokeable cocaine accumulate punishment in their bodies, and their debts steadily increase in that "moral economy of violence" (Karandinos et al. 2014) that is the cocaine base paste market (Albano et al. 2014).

---

[16] These concepts could be useful to think a strategic retreat from the prohibitionist complex. Sunkel (2006) and other Chilean scholars have used them profitably to think about the *market-centric* neoliberal dictatorship in Chile.

[17] https://elpais.com/internacional/2016/09/30/actualidad/1475226573_805987.html

Uruguayan drug policies imply progressive and civilizing protection for integrated subjects through a state-centric form that protects the users of cannabis from the possibility of becoming entrapped by the State in very same violence. As a counterpoise and without showing any fissures, this policy exerts a high punitive pressure over the *pastosos* and *pichis*, to whom it allocates spaces of advanced liberal governmentality where they experience such pressure on a daily basis. In addition, as happens in other areas, the needs of the most vulnerable are catered for by the most precarious workers.

As a result, Uruguayan policy offers a model that does not leave to the market the regulation of the use of substances potentially harmful to health. Furthermore, it confronts the endurance of a prohibition that favors the growth of a violent drug market.

> "With contrasting models in Uruguay versus the Colorado and Washington schemes, there will be much to learn from the first ten years of legal cannabis markets. One wonders whether the second decade will see the triumph of public health over private profit." (Lenton 2014, p. 358)

This contrast expresses two distinct civilizational processes, two mechanisms that are already in motion in order to overcome the damage caused by the War-on-Drugs strategy and, sooner or later, to abandon the dense networks of the prohibitionist complex.[18]

References

Albano, G., Castelli, L., Martínez, E., & Rossal, M. (2015). Violencias institucionales y reproducción de estigmas en usuarios de cocaínas fumables de Montevideo. *Psicologia em Pesquisa, 9*(2), 111–125.

Albano, G., Castelli, L., Martínez, E., & Rossal, M. (2014). Caminando solos. In M. Rossal & H. Suárez (Eds.), *Fisuras. Dos estudios sobre pasta base de cocaína en el Uruguay: Aproximaciones cuantitativas y etnográficas* (pp. 61–148). Montevideo: OUD/JND/FHCE.

Arocena, F., & Aguiar, S. (2017). Tres leyes innovadoras en Uruguay: Aborto, matrimonio homosexual y regulación de la marihuana. *Revista de Ciencias Sociales, 30*(40), 43–62.

Auyero, J., Burbano de Lara, A., & Berti, M. F. (2014). Violence and the state at the urban margins. *Journal of Contemporary Ethnography, 43*(1), 94–116.

Azaola, E. (2012). La violencia de hoy, las violencias de siempre. *Desacatos, 40*, 13–32.

Bardazano, G. (2014). Respuestas estatales a los usuarios de sustancias psicoactivas en Uruguay: entre la alternativa y la profundización de la guerra a las drogas. In C. P. Correa & C. Youngers (Eds.), *En busca de los derechos: Usuarios de drogas y las respuestas estatales en América Latina*. México: CIDE.

Barrán, J. P. (1992). *Medicina y sociedad en el Uruguay del novecientos: El poder de curar*. Montevideo: Banda Oriental.

---

[18] Currently, the prohibitionist complex is showing one of its most effective facets: the financial system. International financial regulations have forced Uruguayan banks to close the accounts of pharmacies that had decided to sell cannabis, making an additional difficulty for the Uruguayan model of regulation of cannabis. http://www.elobservador.com.uy/bancos-privados-empiezan-cerrar-cuentas-empresas-vinculadas-marihuana-n1104674

Becker, G. S., Murphy, K. M., & Grossman, M. (2004). *The economic theory of illegal goods: The case of drugs (working paper 10976)*. Cambridge, MA: National Bureau of Economic Research.
Brumm, H. J., & Cloninger, D. O. (1994). Drug war and the homicide rate: A direct correlation. *Cato Journal, 14*, 509.
Bourdieu, P. (1997). *Razones prácticas. Sobre la teoría de la acción*. Barcelona: Anagrama.
Bourdieu, P. (1999). *La miseria del mundo*. Buenos Aires: FCE.
Bourgois, P. (2009). Treinta años de retrospectiva etnográfica sobre la violencia en las Américas. *Guatemala: violencias desbordadas, 12*, 27–62.
Burkhart, G. (2009). Creencias normativas en estrategias preventivas: una espada de doble fi lo. Efectos de la percepción de normas y normalidad en campañas informativas, programas escolares y medidas ambientales. *Revista Española de Drogodependencias, 34*(4), 376–400.
Caetano, G. (2011). *La república Batllista*. Montevideo: Ediciones de la Banda Oriental.
Castro, G. (2015). Narcotizando la Guerra Fría. Orígenes históricos del control de drogas en Uruguay. *Contemporánea. Historia y problemas del siglo XX, 6*(6), 83–102.
Courtwright, D. T. (2014). Foreword: Drug use and prohibition: Three reform traditions. In B. C. Labate & C. Cavnar (Eds.), *Prohibition, religious freedom, and human rights: Regulating traditional drug use*. Berlin: Springer.
Das, V., & Poole, D. (2004). State and its margins: Comparative ethnographies. In D. Poole & M. C. Ferme (Eds.), *Anthropology in the margins of the state*. New Mexico: School of American Research Press.
Elias, N. (1988). *El proceso de la civilización. Investigaciones sociogenéticas y psicogenéticas*. Buenos Aires: Fondo de Cultura Económica.
Fraiman, R., & Rossal, M. (2011). *De calles, trancas y botones. Una etnografía sobre violencia y solidaridad urbana*. Montevideo: BID/MI.
Friedman, M. (1991). The war we are losing. In M. B. Krauss & E. P. Lazear (Eds.), *Searching for alternatives: Drug-control policy in the United States* (pp. 53–67). Stanford: Hoover Institution Press.
Galaín, P. (2015). ¿Existe un nuevo modelo de regulación jurídica del cannabis? Cuestiones abiertas en el sistema jurídico de Uruguay. *Anatomia do Crime: Revista de Ciencias Jurídico-Criminais, 2*, 55–84.
Goldstein, P. J. (1985). The drugs/violence nexus: A tripartite conceptual framework. *Journal of Drug Issues, 15*(4), 493–506.
Graham, L. (2015). Legalizing marijuana in the shadows of international law: The Uruguay, Colorado, and Washington models. *Wisconsin International Law Journal, 33*, 140–166.
Guigou, N. (2003). *La nación laica: religión civil y mito-praxis en el Uruguay*. Montevideo: Ediciones La Gotera.
Hughes, C. E., & Stevens, A. (2010). What can we learn from the Portuguese decriminalization of illicit drugs? *The British Journal of Criminology, 50*(6), 999–1022.
Karandinos, G., Hart, L. K., Castrillo, F. M., & Bourgois, P. (2014). The moral economy of violence in the US inner city. *Current Anthropology, 55*(1), 1.
Lenton, S. (2014). New regulated markets for recreational cannabis: Public health or private profit? *Addiction, 109*(3), 354–359.
Levine, H. G., & Reinarman, C. (1991). From prohibition to regulation: Lessons from alcohol policy for drug policy. *The Milbank Quarterly, 69*, 461–494.
Loeck, J. (2014). *A dependencia química e seus cuidados. Antropologia de políticas públicas e de experiências de indivíduos em situação terapêutica na cidade de Porto Alegre. RS* (PhD thesis, Antropología Social, UFRGS, Porto Alegre).
Lusane, C., & Desmond, D. (1991). *Pipe dream blues: Racism and the war on drugs*. Boston: South End Press.
Martínez, M. L. (2010). Historia de la producción de carburante nacional en Uruguay. *Llull: Revista de la Sociedad Española de Historia de las Ciencias y de las Técnicas, 33*(72), 289–314.
Martínez Oró, D. P. (2015). Clubs sociales de cannabis: normalización, neoliberalismo, oportunidades políticas y prohibicionismo. *Clivatge. Estudis i testimonis sobre el conflicte i el canvi socials, 3*, 92–112.

Menéndez, E. (1985). Modelo hegemónico, crisis socio-económica y estrategias de acción del sector salud. *Cuadernos Médico Sociales, 33*, 3–34.
Morone, J. A. (1997). Enemies of the people: The moral dimension to public health. *Journal of Health Politics, Policy and Law, 22*(4), 993–1020.
Müller, C., & Draper, G. (2017). *Marihuana oficial. Crónica de un experimento uruguayo.* Montevideo: Sudamericana.
Musto, D. F. (1999). *The American disease: Origins of narcotic control.* Oxford: Oxford University Press.
Negro, C. (2013). La nueva regulación de la pasta base de cocaína. Maldita pasta base. *Revista de Derecho Penal, 21*, 21–34.
Panter-Brick, C. (2002). Street children, human rights, and public health: A critique and future directions. *Annual Review of Anthropology, 31*, 147–171.
Reuter, P. (2009). Systemic violence in drug markets. *Crime, Law and Social Change, 52*(3), 275–284.
Rose, N., O'Malley, P., & Valverde, M. (2012). Gubernamentalidad. *Astrolabio Nueva Época, 8*, 113–152.
Rossal, M., & Suárez, H. (2016). *Viajes sintéticos. Estudios sobre usos de drogas de síntesis en el Uruguay contemporáneo.* Montevideo: OUD/JND/FHCE.
Sapriza, G. (2002). *La utopía eugenista. Raza, sexo y género en las políticas de población en Uruguay (1920-1945)* (Master's thesis, Facultad de Humanidades y Ciencias de la Educación, Montevideo).
Sunkel, O. (2006). En busca del desarrollo perdido. *Problemas del desarrollo, 37*(147), 13–44.
Silva Forné, D. (2016). *Drogas y Derecho Penal en el Uruguay: tolerancia, prohibición, regulación. Evolución del derecho uruguayo, su doctrina y jurisprudencia. Análisis de la Ley de Regulación y Control del Mercado de la Marihuana.* Montevideo: FCU.
Suárez, H., & Ramírez, J. (2014). Los desposeídos. In M. Rossal & H. Suárez (Eds.), *Fisuras. Dos estudios sobre pasta base de cocaína en el Uruguay: aproximaciones cuantitativas y etnográficas* (pp. 23–60). Montevideo: OUD/JND/FHCE.
Thoumi, F. E. (2013). La marihuana recreativa en los estados de Colorado y Washington y la incapacidad del Gobierno de Estados Unidos para hacer cumplir las leyes federales y las convenciones de drogas dentro de su país. *Colombia Internacional, 79*, 219–248.
Vanger, M. I. (1983). *El país modelo: José Batlle y Ordóñez, 1907–1915.* Montevideo: Editorial Arca.
Wacquant, L. (2010). *Castigar a los pobres. El gobierno neoliberal de la inseguridad social.* Barcelona: Gedisa.
Wacquant, L. (2012). Three steps to a historical anthropology of actually existing neoliberalism. *Caderno CRH, 25*(66), 505–518.
Wiseman, S. F. (1985). Communist ideology and the substance abuser: A peripatetic look at the use of the medical paradigm to oppress political deviants. *Journal of Drug Issues, 15*(2), 247–261.

Part II
Social Issues

Chapter 4
Drugs and Poverty: Interfaces of Oppression in the Capitalist World

Verônica Morais Ximenes, Fernando Santana de Paiva, James Ferreira Moura Jr, and Pedro Henrique Antunes da Costa

Abstract The topic of drugs and poverty is part of a discussion that is the reality of Brazil and other countries. These two issues have together had an impact on processes of oppression in people's lives. This chapter aims to discuss the impact and functions of drug use among populations living in poverty. We discuss some misconceptions that occur when linking the structural responsibilities of the capitalist system only to people who experience the naturalization of poverty, blame for their situation, and criminalization of the use of drugs. Discrimination practices develop as a result of stigmatization of social classes and drug use issues, creating humiliation, feelings of shame, and fatalistic behavior. Actions of denaturalization and decriminalization are presented, using a contextualized view of social problems. An analysis of the implications of such practices in the lives of people who go through contexts of poverty and drug use is also presented.

V. M. Ximenes
Universidade Federal do Ceará, Fortaleza, Brazil
e-mail: vemorais@yahoo.com.br

F. S. de Paiva
Universidade Federal de Juiz de Fora, Juiz de Fora, Brazil
e-mail: fernandosantana.paiva@yahoo.com.br

J. F. Moura Jr (✉)
Universidade da Integração Internacional da Lusofonia Afro-Brasileira, Redenção, Ceará, Brazil
e-mail: jamesferreirajr@gmail.com

P. H. A. da Costa
Faculdade Machado Sobrinho, Juiz de Fora, Brazil
e-mail: phantunes.costa@gmail.com

T. M. Ronzani (ed.), *Drugs and Social Context*,
https://doi.org/10.1007/978-3-319-72446-1_4

4.1 Introduction

The topic of poverty has many different views and is conceived in many different ways. It has the capacity of bringing together many different areas of knowledge, public policies, and institutions. As a social problem, poverty has existed since the beginning of humanity and is still present, as well as the phenomenon of drug use/abuse and, more recently, its criminalization. However, the contexts of drug use by people in situations of poverty need to be focused. The contexts of oppression in this chapter are related to people who live in the street and urban peripheries that are dominated by drug traffic. It is important to point out that violence can be symbolic as well as physical, constituting spaces of suffering that affect the body with a real risk of death (Bandeira and Batista 2002).

The use of drugs and specially the abuse of drugs, as well as the scenarios of excess around the production and commercialization of illegal substances, affect the potentiality of being and living and thus compromise the autonomy of individuals. Undoubtedly, poverty, as a concrete reality, aggravates such conditions, which generates a dialectic relationship between drugs and poverty. Taking reality as socially and historically produced, it is necessary to have a clear understanding that there is no linear causal relationship that directs human actions, but rather mediations that need to be understood from the reality that determines them using a psychosocial perspective. From these premises, it is worth questioning in a Brazilian context: Who are the drug users? Where and how do they live? What are the effects of use and abuse on the lives of people living in poverty? How is poverty structured? How is it viewed? In light of the above, this chapter aims to discuss the impacts and functions of drug use among populations living in poverty.

4.2 Views on Poverty and Misconceptions

Many discussions only aim to conduct a monetary analysis of poverty and are limited to the aspect of income and consumer goods. However, from a complex and multidimensional view of poverty, other dimensions need to be incorporated, such as health, education, habitation, nutrition, and subjective implications. The multidimensional poverty perspective requires dialogue with various areas of knowledge in order to become closer to the people living in this situation. According to Sen (2000), poverty is defined as the lack of capacity, which is the impossibility of having access to and choosing what seems most appropriate to their lives. Thus, poverty can be perceived as a state of deprivation of liberty, encompassing both a personal and subjective scope with social, cultural, and structural contexts.

The complexity of the poverty problem leads to an important discussion that focuses on understanding people living in poverty (i.e., the poor). What do they really think? Do they consider themselves poor or not? For Paugam (2007), the subjective focus of poverty is the self-declaration that individuals make about their financial situation and their well-being. The culture of poverty (Lewis 2010) shows common elements that are present in the daily lives of the poor, surpassing specific characteristics of the local, regional, and national contexts. According to Lewis (2010), the culture of poverty is present in the similarity of family structure, in the nature of kinship ties, in consumption patterns, in the sense of community, in the various types of problems, and in aspirations.

This culture of poverty is built within a capitalist system. The economy in this system "is kept in constant flux, both in the search for new markets and by cheaper methods of production and distribution, which guarantee rates of accumulation and increasing profitability" (Mauriel 2011, p. 34). This strengthens the development of rich groups of people who profit, accumulate, and buy a labor force from groups of poor people who sell their labor in a precarious way.

This relationship generates social inequality, which consists of the difference between a small group that holds the profits and a large group that does not have the right to profit from their work. Cimadamore and Cattani (2007) argue that it is impossible to reduce poverty without reducing social inequality, since both are part of the same vicious cycle. For Siqueira (2013, p. 164), "poverty is not a residual, transitory aspect of capitalism, it is structural and a result of its own development. Capitalism generates accumulation in one side, and poverty on the other; neither of them will ever be eliminated." If poverty is structural, it is necessary to understand how it influences and consolidates the life of the poor. Psychology has an important role and can contribute to these discussions by providing a critical view of psychologizing human processes arising from life in conditions of poverty. Ximenes et al. (2016a, b, c) discuss the psychosocial implications of poverty, where the social aspects are related to psychological aspects.

Some problems associated with the processes of oppression and discrimination experienced both by people living in poverty and by drug users can generate assumptions that mistakenly direct the way of seeing and experiencing poverty. Two such assumptions are the naturalization of poverty and that the poor are to blame for their situation. These misconceptions were built and supported for the perpetuation and maintenance of poverty. According to Accorssi, Sacarparo, and Guareschi (Accorssi et al. 2012, p. 537), naturalization is the result of the ideology that is "created when something that is a social and historical creation of humans in a certain historical-social moment, is treated and approached as a natural event." This capitalist and bourgeois ideology is built to favor the processes of apathy and belief in which the immutability of reality rules.

Faced with this challenge, Martín-Baró (2017) attributes to social psychology the objective of examining what is ideological in the human behavior of people and groups that put into use an anti-popular ideology that oppresses, exploits, and provides the processes of passivity, submission, and fatalism.

The understanding of subjective aspects contributes to the deconstruction that poverty is a natural and inevitable phenomenon in which the stronger (rich) outweigh the weaker (poor), something that is given *a priori*, even before birth or choice by poor people. For Siqueira (2013), this conception is related to "Social Darwinism" in which poverty is part of natural selection, whereby the stronger and better biological characteristics determine social relations. The understanding of poverty must be accompanied by analysis of the processes that convert reality into an ideology, in order to denaturalize psychosocial phenomena that reinforce "guilty visions of the poor for their condition and naturalize poverty as an unquestionable fact, always present in humanity" Ximenes et al. (2016a, p. 186).

The other misconception is the premise of blaming the poor for their situation and focusing on the individual processes. These alone generate the guilt for having created the situation of poverty and being responsible for its solution. The burden of responsibility of the individual doubles, and imposes the requirement of individual actions that weaken collective possibilities for coping with the problem of poverty. The dominant discourse is based on individual merit, regardless of whether or not there were the same material conditions and opportunities for all.

Euzébios Filho and Guzzo (2009) show that in capitalist society the poor are seen as being socially devalued and devoid of individual skills, thus imposing blame for their failures, questioning competence, and associating poverty with violence. These ideas and values present in the "ideology of blaming the poor do not serve to explain the limitations of the capitalist model, but to justify social inequality from a supposed individual deficit" (Euzébios Filho and Guzzo 2009, p. 38).

According to Siqueira (2013), this idea of poverty focuses on the dysfunction, pathology, self-responsibility, and culpability of the individual. From this perspective, the poor are people who have chosen to live in poverty, have a mismatch that needs healing, and lack education or training. By characterizing the poor in this way, there is a displacement of the State's accountability and the system of power for an individual who is in a situation of poverty.

From the perspective of blame, Moura Jr. and Ximenes (2016) identify a stigmatized social identity of the poor person that has been built historically by values, representations, prejudices, stigmas, stereotypes, and social roles related to life in poverty. It is not an easy task to break these processes of oppression and domination in which society is structured and impose another way of reading social reality.

4.3 Contexts of Oppression and Psychosocial Implications of Poverty

Livelihoods in poverty are specific and complex. From the perspective of oppression and confrontation, there are a number of factors that cross the trajectory of a poor person. Crenshaw (2002) argues that violence needs to be understood from an intersectional perspective in which a class issue such as poverty can create oppression. If the person is a black woman, poverty also affects gender and race violence. Drug use can be also conceived as a form of oppression, depending on the type of drug and where the individual is positioned in society. However, Bernardino-Costa (2015) indicates that there are also processes of resistance in these marginalized groups and contexts.

It is known that there are several psychosocial implications related specifically to poverty. Psychosocial implications are the blend of broader macrosocial and ideological aspects that influence the individual's psychological state in a dialectic process of constant fusion and conflict (Moura et al. 2014a). The psychosocial implications of poverty cannot be perceived as an overlapping of the social and psychological scopes, but as a continuous construction in which the psyche is structured from a dialectical relation with social, contextual, and cultural factors.

Homelessness is understood as the use of the public space for existence (Mattos and Ferreira 2004). People in this situation use squares, public places, abandoned buildings, and public facilities to stay overnight or for temporary or permanent shelter. People in this situation can be categorized as in extreme poverty with multidimensional deprivations, such as drug abuse, violence, discrimination, and various forms of physical and mental illness (Rosa et al. 2006). Fear, anxiety, and suffering are constant in people who live in the street because of their exposure to physical and social inclemencies. People living in the street are constantly physically and symbolically attacked by police officers, passersby, and even by people in the same situation (Moura et al. 2014b).

In order to understand better how these contextual aspects affect the lives of people living in poverty, psychosocial categories of confrontation and oppression should be considered. In the perspective of confrontation, there is the capacity of human beings to be more, that is, to expand their possibilities of existence by developing a critical awareness (Freire 1980).

However, there are also several psychosocial implications on the level of domination. Processes of humiliation, feelings of shame, fatalism, and psychic illness function in a psychosocial way as a means of maintaining the *status quo*. According to Moura Jr. and Ximenes (2016), society is structured historically in a perspective of stigmatization of poverty. This way, there is a symbolic social universe that constructs policies of regulatory identity for people in situations of poverty based on inferiority characteristics. A number of practices, values, and beliefs define the way of living of the poor, developing a specific form of identity that is "denied, suffered, helpless, fragile, and also violent" (Góis 2005, p. 60).

This stigmatization can foster acts of humiliation against those individuals that are placed on a lower level by the discriminating agent in a vexing public display (Schick 1997). These acts of humiliation can be represented by gestures and words, generating deep suffering and feelings of shame (La Taille 2002). This different humiliation does not necessarily demand an external agent, since it refers to an overall assessment of failure developed by the individual (Zavaleta 2007). In this way, the stigmatizations present in society can constitute a psychosocial form that influences the psyche of the individual (Prilleltensky 2008). Therefore, humiliation and shame can have repercussions such as social and community isolation.

Fatalism may be one of the few strategies of response to a reality of oppressive deprivation (Cidade et al. 2012). According to Martín-Baró (1998), fatalism is divided into ideas, feelings, and behaviors. These are conceived by passivity and conformity. The feelings are based on apathy and an appreciation of suffering as justified by an idea of predestination. Thus, these ideas are the conceptions of a supernatural force as justification for the reality and life trajectory of the individuals in a predestined way.

Therefore, situations of poverty focus specifically on the development of psychosocial implications, being constituted as modes of confrontation and domination. To make this reality even more oppressive, depending on the context, the psychosocial constitutions may also be influenced by different scenarios of poverty. Thus, drug use and abuse can play a central role, both as a mechanism of confrontation against this complex and oppressive reality, and as a tool for maintaining the *status quo* in the stigmatized perspective.

4.4 Drugs and Poverty: Between Criminalization and Care

The relationship established between man and drugs is secular, being part of the social and political history of humanity. Drugs include a wide range of psychoactive substances that have been used in different scenarios and fulfill several functions: leisure and recreation, religious expression and practice, social integration, and even the economic survival of some social groups (Carneiro 2002).

Despite the undeniable presence of drugs in human life, the twentieth century saw the process of criminalization of certain substances, characterized as illicit drugs, arguing the need to extirpate them from the earth through prohibitionism[1] and its repressive logic. The consequence was the creation of a drug war policy, which began in the USA and spread over the globe with harmful effects (violence, homicide, pauperization, criminalization, etc.) on the social organization of numerous peoples and collectivities (Boiteux et al. 2017).

Concerning the consumption of these substances, according to the *World Drug Report*, (UNDOC 2015), the prevalence of drug use remains stable throughout the world. It was estimated that a total of 246 million people (just over 5% of the world's population aged 15–64) made use of illicit drugs in 2013. About 27 million people use drugs at a problematic level, nearly half of whom are users of injectable drugs. Moreover, it was estimated that, by 2013, 1.65 million people who inject drugs would be living with HIV. A significant number of drug users continue to lose their lives prematurely around the world, with an estimated 187,100 drug-related deaths by 2013.

Production, commerce, and drug consumption gradually became subject to control by the so-called democratic states, imposing a logic of punishment and mass incarceration directed especially at the poor produced by the contradictions of capitalism. Wacquant (2015) in his well-known thesis, laid bare the transmutation of the welfare state into the criminal state, especially in the USA, but with represen-

[1] This political orientation started in the early twentieth century and deepened in the 1970s. In 1971, then-US President Richard Nixon declared a "War on Drugs" that soon expanded into the rest of the world. The production, trade, and consumption of illicit drugs came to be seen as extraordinarily dangerous and uncontrollable by regular means, which, according to the heralds of the so-called drug war, should be tackled by stricter, more exceptional, emergency measures, through an actual war. This concept is the expression of prohibitionist politics still in vogue in social reality.

tations in other parts of Europe and even in Latin America. The need for management of these social ills originated in the very heart of the capitalist system, with drugs being an important protagonist in the maintenance and perpetuation of the order. In this way, the prohibitionist discourse, in its nature, carries the conflict of classes, the State being the incorporator of bourgeois standards, reinforcing the maintenance of structures as they are.

In this sense, the noxious and bloody "drug war" is not exactly a war on drugs. As recommended by Karam (2017), as in any war, we observe warlike power directed against people – the producers, traders, and consumers of substances regarded as prohibited. Undoubtedly, not all of them are targets, since the most vulnerable are preferred. The "enemies" in this war are, preferably, the representatives of the subaltern classes: poor, nonwhite, and powerless. As Darcy Ribeiro (2006) warns us, the enemies in Brazil, historically, are those that have been and continue to be exploited, used, hoarded, and unable to live their own destinies and stories.

Therefore, the State's punitive power does not affect all of society in an undifferentiated manner. If the globalization of zero-tolerance policies, such as those of prohibitionism, has transferred the problem of criminality to the moral arena, removing the responsibility of the State to overcome the inequalities generated by capitalism itself, such a strategy is ethnic and classist. The USA is the country with the largest prison population in the world (2.2 million), confirming Wacquant's (2015) thesis, followed by China (1.6 million), Russia (700,000), and Brazil (668,000). According to the Brazilian Ministry of Justice (2014), from 2000 to 2014, the Brazilian prison population increased by more than 200%.

Contributing to this growth, since the enactment of Law 11.343 in 2006 (known as the Drug Law), the number of those imprisoned for drug trafficking in Brazil increased from 31,000 to 164,000. These numbers represent a growth of 520% in eight years. In total, 28% of the prison population results from prohibitionism, anchored by class criteria and racist punishment, resulting in processes of racial and poverty criminalization (Brazilian Ministry of Justice 2014).

In the midst of this conflicting produced reality, the differentiation between user and trafficker employed by the Brazilian legislation should use objective criteria such as the amount carried and apprehend at the time of the offense. However, there is no clear definition in the normative-legal apparatus regarding the amount that defines a user or a drug dealer. What prevails are the subjective criteria of the officer or legal operator responsible for judgment of the case. Furthermore, the minimum punishment for drug trafficking was increased, which resulted in an increase in the levels of incarceration in Brazil (Boiteux and Pádua 2012) and the USA (Wacquant 2015).

In this direction, as Karam (2017) warns, the implementation of these practices results in the following: (1) class selectivity in law enforcement (for the poor the legal discourse, for users of economically privileged classes, the medical discourse); (2) concretization of a medical-legal discourse and the possible transition to a falsely sanitarian model that opens the door to segregation and hospitalization, often against the will of drug users. All of this culminates in pathologization, with a fantasy of care that distorts the reality in which these people are inserted.

From this perspective, it is imperative to consider the drug issue not only as a health issue, although it is commonly considered and treated as a "public health issue." Harm reduction appears in this scenario as a rationality that should guide care, aiming to break off the history of segregation and violation of human rights feigned as treatment. Therefore, it uses the principle that drug use is not necessarily a harmful or dangerous practice.

In general, we need to understand the contexts and the structures that surround us (conditions of poverty, ethnic/racial differences, gender, etc.) dialectically, with the specificities existing in the subjects and their relationship with drugs, with the idea that abstinence is not the only possible and desirable outcome. Thus, it is conceivable to foster a logic of care that is not reduced to drugs and does not take abstinence as a prerequisite, excluding, penalizing, and/or blaming those who do not fit this perspective. This way, it is possible to minimize vulnerabilities associated with the use of drugs or to promote better living conditions to potentiate other dimensions through an integrated approach, understanding the individuals beyond drugs (Machado and Boarini 2013).

Poverty affects individuals and collectivities differently when understood in its multidimensionality, articulated to the complexity wrapped around the production, commercialization, and consumption of drugs. Consequently, punitive and hygienist practices (anchored in moralistic, biomedical, and positivist precepts, sponsored by the war and pharmaceutical industries) produce a state of exception, a true abduction and genocide, which are functional and at the disposition of the economic and political system.

4.5 Drugs, Different Subjects, and Poverty as a Concrete Reality in Brazil

The Brazilian National Secretariat on Drug Policies (SENAD) with the Oswaldo Cruz Foundation (FIOCRUZ) conducted a study in 2014 with the aim of outlining the profile of the Brazilian population that uses crack. The study showed that the predominant users of crack in Brazil are young adults with an average age of 30 years. Also, they are predominantly male (60%), with a predominance of "non-white" people (80%). Most (55%) reported dropping out of school during their elementary education (Bastos and Bertoni 2014).

According to the same study, approximately 40% of crack users in the country and 47% in the capitals were homeless. Because they have developed social practices that are considered "deviant," to which are attributed great social costs, these users distance themselves from the values and rules considered socially accepted by the "majority" of people in society. Consequently, they live with stigmas and violence inherent to such "deviations," resulting in separation and confinement of this group in a limited urban space, without interaction with the nearest residents, except those under similar conditions (Vallim et al. 2015).

As expected, this situation is followed by marginalization and reinforcement of social practices of stigmatization and social humiliation. These practices strengthen behaviors considered inadequate, which culminate in the deepening of prejudice and social oppression. As these individuals are usually associated with drug use and dependence, the stigmas generated in the social imagery regarding their lives become more intense (Dantas et al. 2012). In the street context, the use of drugs, more precisely crack, is assimilated with the stigma of the homeless, who historically carry representations of the dangers associated with poverty, materialized in the idea of dangerous classes, as discussed by Coimbra (2007) in order to identify enemies of the established order.

The stigma of drug use is used as a further strategy of depreciation, guilt, and penalty for the condition experienced, constituting an ideological strategy of domination and differentiation of power that contributes to the maintenance of the social abyss still in force (Parker and Aggleton 2001). "The result is the production of the social identity of the 'drunkard,' that is, trickster, drunk, which disqualifies these people and guides how to treat them" (Alcântara et al. 2015, p. 5), denying them diverse possibilities of existence and reducing their identity to this unique form of recognition (Moura and Ximenes 2016).

In this direction, poverty combined with drug consumption develops a social identity, highlighted by disqualification (Paugam 2003) and full of ethical-political suffering (Sawaia 2006) for these individuals. Discrimination practices develop because of the combined stigmatization of class and drug use issues, which generates acts of humiliation, feelings of shame, and fatalistic behavior (Moura et al. 2014b). The meanings attributed to the use of drugs are different for the homeless population, and it is crucial that we do not analyze the drug as a problem per se, because it is a challenge among so many other problems found on the street.

It is dangerous to believe in the commonly held sense, supported by media discourses, that only drugs lead people to live and/or stay on the streets. This ideology also has repercussions on family and social relationships marked by these forms of stigmatized recognition (Moura and Ximenes 2016). These analyses only legitimize ideological precepts of blaming the subjects for socially and economically constituted ills. In a context of extreme poverty such as that symbolized by the street situation, analysis of the implications of drug use seems more complex: After all, what do we consider as problematic consumption in the life of those who are hungry, cold, and sleep on the street?

From this perspective, Rui (2006) believes that drug use may be better understood if we demarcate the markers of social class as crucial for advancing analyses and interventions. Social hierarchies are expressed in the dynamics of drug use, with legitimation of those who can and do have control over whether or not to use these substances. In addition, access to knowledge and even care is diametrically different when we consider the poverty dimension as a condition of differentiation of subjects.

Also, regarding the context of drug use in homeless situations, we would like to point out that women are in a situation characterized by greater oppression and vulnerability to human rights violations due to historical gender inequalities that are still present in our social reality. Gender is a category that also refers to the issues of identity and subjectivity and is constructed with reference to a particular model of society, with delimited patterns of what is male and female. This is guided by a patriarchal structure that places men and women in a hierarchy, inherent in the beginnings of the social and sexual division of labor (Cortina 2015).

Regarding homeless women, we observe a set of situations, such as maternity and different types of violence (physical and psychological), in addition to the usual cases of sexual abuse and beatings, which are strengthened by the recurrent stigmas and prejudices around the status of women and affect their social identity (Lopes et al. 2003). Regarding the use of crack by women, the FIOCRUZ study found a series of differences linked to the gender asymmetries in our society, such as greater frequency of use (average of 21 crack rocks a day, compared with 13 for men); higher percentage of subjects involved in prostitution (29.9% against 1.3% of men); and higher prevalence of sexual violence (44.5%) than men (7.0%) who, first and foremost, are the perpetrators of this type of gender oppression (Bastos and Bertoni 2014).

According to Cortina (2015) in a study about women and drug trafficking, the entrance of poor women into the drug trade occurs due to the well-known feminization of poverty (Lavinas et al. 2012). This is expressed in different situations: (1) difficulties in supporting children alone; (2) barriers in the process of insertion in the work market, given their low education and lack of the professional training demanded by the liberal-bourgeois market. In the case of women who use drugs and live in street situations, we have the conformation of a framework of wide oppression, which imposes on these subjects a condition of sub-citizenship, also expressing the social abyss that exists in Brazil and other countries around the globe.

We also experience the acknowledged genocide against poor and black youths living in peripheries of urban centers, who are the main targets of homicides, both as victims and victimizers (Barros et al. 2008). A young black man in Brazil is 2.4 times more likely to be murdered, and homicide is among the leading causes of unnatural violent death among young people (Presidency of the Republic 2015).

The relationship between these data and the scenario of production, commerce, and use of drugs is widely recognized, culminating in disastrous effects on the life of this specific youth segment. Regarding consumption, a discourse of alleged "democratization" has emerged, creating an idea that drugs are part of and afflict the lives of all young people, based on a trans-classist and decontextualized logic. This discourse aims to obscure the capacity for analysis and understanding of the reality experienced by vulnerable and oppressed young people from the suburbs. As a result, we observe once again selectivity as a way of understanding the social dynamics: the medical stereotype is always applied to the middle-class young people, who are in fact the biggest drug users, and the criminal stereotype is applied to the young poor people who sell it (Batista 2003; Karam 2017).

As pointed out by Góes (2008), in the midst of the cyclical and structural crisis of capitalism, disguised as modernization and a technological revolution, we observe a large contingent of young people who do not participate in the capitalist production process, as they are not formally registered in the middle-class labor market and serve as an industrial reserve army. The other way out for this population contingent, already highlighted above, is extermination. The black and young poor people (representatives of the subaltern classes) are conceived as superfluous; at the same time, they are functional for the perpetuation of this unequal social order, which is materialized by the State and its repressive arm. In this sense, a true hunt is carried out with the refinements and strategies of war, ideologically built to manage drugs, especially regarding the production and commercialization considered illegal in the social sphere; in short, an efficient strategy of arresting, killing. and silencing.

4.6 Final Considerations

This chapter analyzes the functions and impacts of drugs in the lives of people living in poverty. It considers that both drugs and poverty should be seen as expressions of a societal order that is, in principle, contradictory and marked by social inequalities. This scenario is complex in that the responses offered by the State, in the form of public policies, perpetuate the logic of segregation, repression, and criminalization and, on the other hand, provide assistance that is sometimes precarious and crossed by moralistic and stigmatizing practices.

Therefore, to change and overcome this complex picture, it is imperative that we employ comprehensive analytical efforts, considering the vicissitudes and multifaceted nature of the reality, in order to develop ways for effective social transformation. In this case, it is essential to overcome poverty as a condition that supports the current capitalist project, as well as take a realistic view of the relationship between man and drugs, which means adopting a policy of legalization of all drugs and suppressing prohibitionism. Thus, it will be possible to avoid and at the same time challenge perspectives that consider poverty and drugs in a simplistic way and, above all, to challenge those who use this perspective to maintain the *status quo*.

References

Accorssi, A., Scarparo, H., & Guareschi, P. (2012). A naturalização da pobreza: reflexões sobre a formação do pensamento social. *Psicologia & Sociedade, 24*(3), 536–546. https://doi.org/10.1590/S0102-71822012000300007.

Alcântara, S. C., Abreu, D. P., & Farias, A. A. (2015). Pessoas em situação de rua: das trajetórias de exclusão social aos processos emancipatórios de formação de consciência, identidade e sentimento de pertença. *Revista Colombiana de Psicología, 24*(1), 129–143.

Bandeira, L., & Batista, A. S. (2002). Preconceito e Discriminação como expressões da violência. *Estudos Feministas, 10*, 119–141.

Barros, N. V., Moreira, C. A., & Duarte, K. M. (2008). Juventude e criminalização da pobreza. *Educere et Educare: Revista em Educação, 3*(5), 141–148.

Bastos, F. I., & Bertoni, N. (2014). *Pesquisa Nacional sobre o uso do crack: quem são os usuários de crack e/ou similares do Brasil? Quantos são nas capitais brasileiras?* Rio de Janeiro: Editora ICICT/FIOCRUZ.

Batista, V. M. (2003). *Difíceis ganhos fáceis: Drogas e juventude pobre no Rio de Janeiro*. Rio de Janeiro: Revan.
Bernardino-Costa, J. (2015). Decolonialidade e interseccionalidade emancipadora: a organização política das trabalhadoras domésticas no Brasil. *Sociedade e Estado, 30*(1), 147–163.
Boiteux, L., Chernicharo, L. P., & Alves, C. S. (2017). Direitos humanos e convenções internacionais de drogas: Em busca de uma razão humanitária nas leis de drogas. In M. Dalla Vecchia, T. M. Ronzani, F. S. Paiva, C. B. Batista, & P. H. A. Costa (Eds.), *Drogas e Direitos Humanos: Reflexões em Tempos de Guerra às Drogas* (pp. 233–264). Porto Alegre: Rede Unidade.
Boiteux, L., & Pádua, J. P. (2012). La desproporción de la Ley de Drogas: los costes humanos y económicos de la actual política en Brasil. In C. P. Correa (Ed.), *Justicia desmedida: Proporcionalidad y delitos de drogas en America Latina* (pp. 71–101). Ciudad de Mexico: Fontamara.
Brazilian Ministry of Justice. (2014). *Levantamento nacional de informações penitenciárias (INFOPEN)*. Brasília: Ministério da Justiça.
Carneiro, H. (2002). As necessidades humanas e o proibicionismo das drogas no século XX. *Outubro, 6*, 115–128.
Cidade, E. C., Moura, J. F., Jr., & Ximenes, V. M. (2012). Implicações Psicológicas da Pobreza na Vida do povo Latino-Americano. *Psicologia Argumento, 30*(68), 58–75.
Cidamore, A., & Cattani, D. (2007). A construção da pobreza e da desigualdade na América Latina: uma introdução. In A. Cidamore & D. Cattani (Eds.), *Produção de pobreza e desigualdade na América Latina* (pp. 7–14). Porto Alegre: Tomo.
Coimbra, C. M. B. (2007). Direitos humanos e criminalização da pobreza. In S. M. Freire (Ed.), *Direitos humanos: violência e pobreza na América Latina contemporânea* (pp. 130–144). Rio de Janeiro: Letra e Imagem.
Cortina, M. O. C. (2015). Mulheres e tráfico de drogas: aprisionamento e criminologia feminista. *Revista Estudos Feministas, 23*(3), 761–778.
Crenshaw, K. (2002). Documento para o Encontro de Especialistas em Aspectos da Discriminação Racial Relativos ao Gênero. *Estudos Feministas, 10*, 171–188.
Dantas, B. S. A., Turibio, M. T. M., Atanes, R. T., & Almeida, R. S. (2012). Políticas Públicas sobre Drogas e População de Rua: humanização ou coisificação dos sujeitos? *Revista Gestão & Políticas Públicas, 2*(2).
Euzébios Filho, A., & Guzzo, R. (2009). Desigualdade social e pobreza: contexto de vida e de sobrevivência. *Psicologia & Sociedade, 21*(1), 35–44.
Freire, P. (1980). *Conscientização: teoria e prática da libertação—uma introdução ao pensamento de Paulo Freire* (3rd ed.). São Paulo: Cortez e Moraes.
Góis, C. W. L. (2005). *Psicologia Comunitária: atividade e consciência*. Fortaleza: Publicações Instituto Paulo Freire de Estudos Psicossociais.
Góes, W. L. (2008). Genocídio da juventude negra: da acumulação primitiva a superfluidade. *BIS. Boletim do Instituto de Saúde (Impresso), 44*, 23–25.
Karam, M. L. (2017). Considerações sobre as políticas criminais, drogas e direitos humanos. In M. Dalla Vecchia, T. M. Ronzani, F. S. Paiva, C. B. Batista, & P. H. A. Costa (Eds.), *Drogas e Direitos Humanos: Reflexões em Tempos de Guerra às Drogas* (pp. 211–232). Porto Alegre: Rede Unidade.
La Taille, Y. (2002). *Vergonha: a ferida moral*. Petrópolis: Vozes.
Lavinas, L., Cobo, B., & Veiga, A. (2012). Bolsa Família: impacto das transferências de renda sobre a autonomia das mulheres pobres e as relações de gênero. *Revista Latinoamericana de Población, 10*(6), 31–56.
Lewis, O. (2010). *Antropologia de la pobreza: cinco famílias* (24th ed.). México: FCE. First published in Spanish in 1961.
Lopes, R. E., Borba, P. L. O., & Reis, T. A. M. (2003). Um olhar sobre as trajetórias, percursos e histórias de mulheres em situação de rua. *Cadernos de Terapia Ocupacional da UFSCar, 2*(1), 39–52.
Machado, L. V., & Boarini, M. L. (2013). Políticas sobre drogas no Brasil: a estratégia de redução de danos. *Psicologia: Ciência e Profissão, 33*(3), 580–593.

Martín-Baró, I. (1998). *Psicología de la liberación*. Madrid, España: Trotta.
Martín-Baró, I. (2017). A desideologização como contribuição da Psicologia Social para o desenvolvimento da democracia na América Latina. In I. Martín-Baró (Ed.), *Crítica e libertação na Psicologia: estudos psicossociais*. Petrópolis, RJ: Vozes. First published in 1985.
Mattos, R. M., & Ferreira, R. F. (2004). Quem vocês pensam que (elas) são? Representações sobre as pessoasem situação de rua. *Psicologia & Sociedade, 16*(2), 47–58.
Mauriel, A. (2011). *Capitalismo, políticas sociais e combate à pobreza*. Ijuí, RS: Editora Unijuí.
Moura, J. F., Jr., Cidade, E. C., Ximenes, V. M., & Sarriera, J. C. (2014a). Concepções de pobreza: um convite à discussão psicossocial. *Temas em Psicologia (Ribeirão Preto), 22*, 341–352.
Moura, J. F., Jr., Ximenes, V. M., & Sarriera, J. C. (2014b). Práticas de discriminação às pessoas em situação de rua: histórias de vergonha, de humilhação e de violência em Fortaleza, Brasil. *Revista de Psicología, 22*, 18–28.
Moura, J. F., Jr., & Ximenes, V. M. (2016). A identidade social estigmatizada de pobre: uma constituição opressora. *Fractal: Revista de Psicologia, 28*(1), 76–83.
Parker, R., & Aggleton, P. (2001). *Estigma, discriminação e Aids*. Rio de Janeiro: Coleção ABIA. Cidadania e Direitos.
Paugam, S. (2003). *Desqualificação social: ensaio sobre a nova pobreza*. São Paulo: Educ/Cortez.
Paugam, S. (2007). *Las formas elementales de la pobreza*. Madrid: Alianza Editorial.
Presidency of the Republic. (2015). *Índice de vulnerabilidade juvenil à violência e desigualdade racial 2014*. Brasília: Presidência da República.
Prilleltensky, I. (2008). The role of power in wellness, oppression, and liberation: the promise of psychopolitical validity. *Journal of Community Psychology, 36*(2), 116–136.
Ribeiro, D. (2006). *O povo brasileiro: A formação e o sentido do Brasil*. São Paulo: Companhia das Letras.
Rosa, A. S., Secco, M. G., & Brêttas, A. C. P. (2006). O cuidado emsituação de rua: revendo o significado do processo de saúde-doença. *Revista Brasileira de Enfermagem, 59*(3), 331–336.
Rui, T. C. (2006). Só se vive uma vez: uma reflexão acerca de distintas concepções e práticas do uso de "drogas". *Revista Mediações, 11*(2), 187–202.
Sawaia, B. B. (2006). *As artimanhas da exclusão: uma análise ético-psicossocial da desigualdade*. Petrópolis: Vozes.
Schick, F. (1997). On humiliation. *Social Research, 64*(1), 131–138.
Sen, A. (2000). *Desenvolvimento como liberdade*. São Paulo: Companhia das Letras.
Siqueira, L. (2013). *Pobreza e serviço social: diferentes concepções e compromissos políticos*. São Paulo: Cortez Editora.
UNODC. (2015). *World drug report*. New York: United Nations Office on Drugs and Crime (UNODC).
Vallim, D. C., Zaluar, A., & Sampaio, C. (2015). Uma etnografia das cenas de uso de crack no Rio de Janeiro e seus efeitos nos usuários. In M. Teixeira & Z. Fonseca (Eds.), *Saberes e práticas na atenção primária à saúde: cuidado à população em situação de rua e usuários de álcool, crack e outras drogas* (pp. 201–216). São Paulo: Hucitec.
Wacquant, L. (2015). *Punir os pobres: a nova gestão da miséria nos Estados Unidos*. Rio de Janeiro: Revan.
Ximenes, V., Nepomuceno, B., & Cidade, E. (2016a). Pobreza: um problema para a Psicologia Comunitária? In V. Ximenes, J. Sarriera, Z. Bomfim, & J. Alfaro (Eds.), *Psicologia Comunitária no mundo atual: desafios, limites e fazeres* (pp. 175–196). Fortaleza: Expressão Gráfica e Editora.
Ximenes, V., Nepomuceno, B., Cidade, E., & Moura Júnior, J. F. (2016b). *Implicações Psicossociais da Pobreza: diversidades e resistências*. Fortaleza: Expressão Gráfica e Editora.
Ximenes, V. M., Moura, J. F., Jr., Cruz, J. M., Silva, L. B., & Sarriera, J. C. (2016c). Pobreza multidimensional e seus aspectos subjetivos em contextos rurais e urbanos nordestinos. *Estudos de Psicologia, 21*(2), 146–156.
Zavaleta, D. R. (2007). The Ability to go About Without Shame: A Proposal for Internationally Comparable Indicators. *Working Paper 03 OPHI*. Oxford Poverty & Human Development Initiative, OPHI.

Chapter 5
Drugs and Gender

Nuria Romo-Avilés

Abstract Gender construction is performative and creates fundamental differences in drug use and abuse. Women tend to consume drugs that are licit and socially accepted to a greater degree than men. This has made them invisible in the world of drug dependence. In recent decades, they have been moving more and more towards consuming typically masculine drugs. However, when they consume illegal drugs, particularly in contexts of social exclusion, they are subject to processes of social stigmatization and rejection. Women suffer situations of violence associated with their drug consumption, they are being affected by their participation in the lowest levels of drug trafficking, and they have fewer possibilities of receiving treatment or benefitting from preventative programmes adapted to their needs. From an intersectional perspective, it is important to take age, ethnicity, religious beliefs and other variables that interact with gender into account. Looking through gender creates a new view: it changes some of the key concepts of drug dependence, such as addiction, but above all it generates the possibility of designing drug policies sensitive to male and female users, open to the regulation of substance consumption, and more understanding and respectful of the rights of the men and women who consume drugs.

5.1 Drugs and Gender: Tools for a New Understanding of Drug Abuse

Imagine a day like any other, leaving your house or work; you come across a person passed out due to the effects of taking some kind of psychoactive substance or drug. Would your thoughts be the same whether you identified them as a woman or as a

The data presented here form part of the project entitled "Gender and interpersonal violence in the recreational contexts of adolescent free time". R+D+I Projects of the State Plan of Technical and Scientific Research. Spanish Ministry of Economy, Industry and Competitiveness. (Reference FEM2016-77116-C2-1-R).

N. Romo-Avilés (✉)
Departamento de Antropología Social, Instituto Universitario de Investigación de Estudios de las Mujeres y de Género. Universidad de Granada, Granada, Spain
e-mail: nromo@ugr.es

T. M. Ronzani (ed.), *Drugs and Social Context*,
https://doi.org/10.1007/978-3-319-72446-1_5

man? Would they be able to solve their problems associated with drug abuse in the same way, depending on the sexual identification you make?

We have never known much about the influence of sexual identity for people who use and abuse drugs because drug-dependence studies focus on male experience and neglect others with different heteronormative or non-heteronormative sexual identities. We know that studies on gender and drugs as a research field in public health have barely been developed or disseminated (Llort et al. 2013). Regarding gender perspective, it has been shown how most studies that have been carried out have concealed the experiences, feelings and actions of women in relation to their health and drug consumption (Romo 2010).

Applying gender perspective to drug dependence means visibilizing the process of social construction that generates the social and cultural stereotypes that every society assigns to the behaviour, characteristics and values that are attributed to men and women, and that symbols, laws and regulations, institutions and social perceptions reaffirm in daily life. Behind these stereotypes lies the idea that such characteristics are natural or intrinsic and, therefore, unalterable. Gender is constructed upon the basis of cultural, economic, ethnic, religious, historical and ideological factors, which entail social, economic and political inequalities, in which the activities of men or the activities identified as masculine are perceived as superior in most cultures.

Gender is a learned cultural fact that establishes different mandates. These "gender mandates" determine the different attributes that "Woman and Man" must have, through the constructions of what is femininity and masculinity. For example, the gender mandates in sexuality are rendered into the fulfilment of what the symbolic order establishes as what should be – what is expected of women and what is expected of men. In contemporary European societies, activities that involve risk are within the mandate of masculinity. When a woman consumes illegal drugs, she breaks her gender mandate and creates a rupture with the roles that have been socially and culturally assigned to her, such as that of maternity. For this reason, every time that women use illegal drugs and break the limits of what has been socially imposed by the patriarchy, a social sanction is generated, a rejection caused by breaking the roles assigned to them and disrupting controls on the sexual behavior of women.

I understand "gender" as a theoretical perspective, but also methodological. Gender, however, does not have women or women's roles as its object of study. Gender perspective works with the different forms in which sexual identities are constructed. Gender is a constitutive element of social relations based on the differences that distinguish the sexes and end up causing inequality. Including gender perspective is a key factor in understanding people's attitudes and behaviours regarding drug consumption and its consequences.

For Virginia Maquieira, gender is the structure that crosses socio-structural determinations such as class, age, position in the world order and sexual option. In this way, gender works as a structuring principle of human societies, differentiating between men and women, and converting these differences into hierarchical and unequal relations. In this construction, the culture that legitimates, under its protection, the social relations of disadvantage and oppression towards women; that promulgates the defense of cultural difference, contrasting it with that of gender equality; and that interprets any change in women as a threat to cultural identity and traditions, is deeply implicated (Maqueira 2006).

Gender is a performative notion (Buttler 2007), in which femininities and masculinities are continually (re-)created within local "communities of practice" (Paechter 2003). Connell (2012) maintains that what it is to be a woman or a man within a particular localized community is learned. "From this perspective, gender delimits, defines and expresses, rather, a social position that has the function of constructing individuals historically into 'men' and into 'women' by a process of subjective appropriation of its rules and representations. Gender expresses hierarchical differences between the male and the female, but also produces them through its discourses on Difference".

In the area of public health, the inclusion of gender perspective has brought about a revolutionary examination of the processes of health and illness. For the World Health Organization, "the concept of gender refers to the stereotypes, social roles, acquired condition and position, appropriate behaviours, activities and attributes that every society in particular constructs and assigns to men and women. All of them can lead to inequalities and, at the same time, these inequalities can cause inequity between men and women, in state of health and right to health" (WHO 2009).

Even though gender analysis is aware of the inequalities between men and women, both in health and drug consumption, this sole analytical category has proved insufficient. Different studies (McCall 2005; Simien 2007; Bowleg 2012) have highlighted how neither women nor men form homogeneous groups and that the heterogeneity within them shows different inequalities.

The concept of intersectionality provides a theoretical and methodological framework that is complementary to that of gender. Analysis that is both intergender and intragender is needed to reveal the inequalities to us. Other analytical categories that structure society, such as social class, ethnicity, sexual orientation, age or religion contribute to generating experiences of oppression, inequality or privilege (Mahalingam et al. 2008). Intersectionality proposes that ethnic group, social class, gender and age are categories that generate socially constructed inequalities, and that interact simultaneously, forming interdependent, intertwining patterns (Crenshaw 1991).

We know that gender conditions exposure and vulnerability to health risk factors. Although protecting factors such as greater awareness and risk prevention are attributed to women, along with greater dedication to self-care, other gender conditions affect their health. The greater burden of caring for other people, above all due to the unequal workload in the domestic sphere, inequalities in access to employment, inequities in salaries and the greater pressure on personal image, among other things, are vulnerability factors for women when it comes to taking care of their health. Moreover, age, social class and education are axes of inequality that interact with gender, producing greater disparity in the health of men and women (García-Calvente et al. 2008).

In order to clarify the possible connection of gender perspective with the world of drug dependence, we must begin to reflect upon the invisibility of women, their choices and needs, and their position in the history of drug policies and in drug dependence in modern-day societies. In this regard, it is essential to understand that considering certain psychoactive substances as a social problem forms part of a historical process that started at the end of the nineteenth century when state interventionist politics began (Romo et al. 2014).

In the mid-nineteenth century, the first attempt to regulate psychoactive substance consumption came about when the expansion of opium use in China and its consequent prohibition by the emperor led to the declaration of two wars by the British, known as the Opium Wars. In 1914, the Harrison Narcotic Law was enacted in the USA to ban the use of narcotics without medical prescription, leading to the subsequent criminalization of certain psychoactive substances in that country and around the world (Márkez Alonso 2010). It was at that time that the boundaries between legal and illegal substances were established, which have lasted until today. Some opiates that had been widely used with legality and above all by women (Kandall 2010) crossed over definitively into illegality. Historical studies have shown how women were opiate consumers in the period when they were legal and could be acquired at chemists' and general stores (Kandall 2010). At the moment when certain substances are considered illegal, women turn to legal and socially accepted drugs, frequently in tandem with the processes of medicalization.

Then heroin appeared, a substance more powerful than morphine, administered intravenously, which in the West caused a whole series of negative consequences associated with the method of administration and not only with the substance itself. Since then, the consumption of illegal psychoactive substances has become a risk behaviour and, as such, is expected of men but not of women. Gender is thus one element more in the construction of illegal drug consumption as a "social problem."

Since that time, differentiation between legal and illegal drugs has become the main way of explaining differences between psychoactive substances, with little attention paid to other characteristics, such as the damage their consumption might inflict on the health of populations. The legality of a substance is determined by the way in which it is used rather than by its health effects. For instance, despite the severe individual and public health problems caused by tobacco and alcohol, these substances remain legal.

In the same way that risk behaviour is considered a part of masculine culture, so is drug dependence. The androcentric positions that have dominated the relevant literature have masked the social construction of the legal or illegal character of psychoactive substances that took place throughout the nineteenth and twentieth centuries. From the beginnings of the construction of the "drug problem." it has been associated with illegality and masculinity. In contrast, women have generally consumed socially accepted drugs and medicines, explaining in part the tendency for females to be ignored in public policymaking on drug dependence (Kandall 2010).

This model of drug policy has failed in the regulation of consumption, in the harm reduction, and in the treatment of people in the world who have become addicts for different reasons (Romo-Avilés, N., 2011). Below, I highlight aspects that show drug policies' lack of sensitivity towards the needs of women, which I will develop in the ensuing sections of this chapter.

- There are differences in the prevalence of drug consumption between men and women and these are not visible in public policies on drug dependence. Women frequently use and abuse legal drugs and suffer from processes of medicalization in different moments of their lives.
- Women suffer from vulnerabilities related to gender inequality, which lead them to become victims of violence. They suffer different types of violence associated with drug abuse and they suffer from the negative consequences of the illegal drug market to a greater degree than men, with a significant increase in recent years in the number of women jailed for minor crimes of drug micro-trafficking around the world.
- Public policies on drugs have no gender sensitivity, in the treatment programmes or prevention and harm-reduction programmes, to the differences and inequalities that exist between people from an intersectional perspective.

5.1.1 Gender Differences in the Use and Abuse of Drugs: Do Men and Women Consume the Same Drugs?

Men are more likely than women to use almost all types of illicit drugs (SAMHSA 2014), and illicit drug use is more likely to result in emergency department visits or overdose deaths for men than for women. This global trend occurs in different countries, but it does not mean that women "do not consume drugs", rather that they tend to lean towards the consumption of licit substances.

In general, "men are three times more likely than women to use cannabis, cocaine or amphetamines, whereas women are more likely than men to engage in the non-medical use of opioids and tranquilizers. Gender disparities in drug use are more attributable to opportunities to use drugs in a social environment than to either gender being more or less susceptible or vulnerable to the use of drugs" (UNODC 2016). In Spain, for example, the latest epidemiological data for young people indicate that women consume fewer illegal drugs than men, but more legal and psychoactive drugs in all age groups, and tobacco and alcohol at younger ages (DGPNSD 2016).

This leads one to believe that the use of illegal drugs among women carries emotional baggage of distaste and fear of it being public, perhaps due to their still predominant role in our societies as dependent wife and caregiving mother (Klee 2001). For women, using an illegal substance entails not only being classified as deviants for their use of drugs, but also for going against the social definition of what "feminine" behaviour should be (Ettorre 1992). Even among drug users, women incite rejection, reporting their preference for "drug-free" female partners.

In recent decades, two epidemiological trends in relation to drug consumption stand out from the point of view of gender. On the one hand, a reduction in the gender gap in the consumption of some drugs and, on the other hand, an increase in some countries in the consumption of all legal substances by the young.

In countries with a long history of drug use, the gender gap in consumption has reduced (OAS and CICAD 2011). Although illicit drug consumption is far higher among men, the gender gap decreases to almost nothing in the case of adolescents, for whom the pattern is mostly associated with recreational motivations (Calafat et al. 2009). Similarly, the latest report by the United Nations indicates that although most studies show that the prevalence of drug consumption is higher in young people that in adults, the gender differences in terms of consumption are lower among the young than among adults (UNODC 2016). This means that women's roles are getting closer to traditional male roles, reflected, for example, in a greater assumption of risk behaviours concerning health. The new models of socialization also appear to be bringing about greater autonomy for women, independence and participation in resources and public life; these are positive advances towards gender equality.

The second trend concerns the increase in the consumption of legal drugs at younger ages. In Spain, for example, since the 1990s, young women appear to have overtaken young men in the consumption of legal drugs (tobacco, alcohol and non-prescribed tranquilizers). According to the most recent school survey by the Spanish Drug Observatory, a higher proportion of girls than boys aged between the ages of 14 and 18 consumed alcohol and tobacco. In addition, non-prescribed tranquilizers were used by 3% of girls in this age group, compared to only 1.8% of boys. In contrast, there was no gender difference in consumption of cannabis, the most prevalent illegal drug among Spanish adolescents (DGPNSD 2010, 2015).

Another of the most striking tendencies in recent decades is concerning the change of trend in the patterns of alcohol consumption, above all in heavy consumption by women. For example, in the case of Argentina, in the latest study by SEDRONAR (2017), the latest epidemiological data reveal an increase in the risky consumption of alcohol by women. In 2010, 6.1% of women between the ages of 12 and 65 consumed alcohol in a manner that was risky and harmful for their health. Today, that figure has risen to 9%, equivalent to 567,285 women.

In the case of Spain, the latest epidemiological data from the National Drugs Plan (Plan Nacional sobre Drogas; PNSD), which funds this research, underlines that 82% of adolescents between the ages of 14 and 18 had consumed alcohol in the last year, with consumption being more widespread among girls, particularly in relation to patterns of heavy drinking. It is no wonder that between 14 and 16 years old the percentage of girls that get drunk is higher than for boys. To understand these aspects, we need to analyse the sociocultural variables that influence risk behaviours in a general way in the use and abuse of recreational substances. The results of this study show that women identify alcohol more and more as a constituent part of their social lives and of their incorporation to certain leisure spaces, which, at least in part, can explain the changes of trend. Nevertheless, previous research shows that differences in metabolism mean that girls are considered more vulnerable to the toxic effects of alcohol. Heavy drinking can have a series of harmful effects on their health, such as liver problems (Romo-Avilés et al. 2016, b).

From this perspective, to assume that gender influences alcohol consumption means that it can be described as a form of "doing gender" (Measham 2002). This frames a key issue of socio-cultural order: women are redefining their gender identities in relation to men through alcohol consumption. However, girls who drink tend to be socially represented as sexually promiscuous and with a higher probability of getting involved in sexual practices of risk: it could mean that the problems derived from consuming alcohol from an early age are minimised or ignored. "Drinking like a boy" can be related to the idea of "transformative empowerment" and/or, in a parallel way, can act as a factor that contributes to strengthen certain vulnerabilities, such as increasing the cases of unwanted sexual relations and exposure to situations of micro-sexism that increase their future vulnerability to situations of gender violence.

We know that in many different countries, sedatives and hypnotics are some of the drugs most consumed by women. It is important to emphasise that distinction between licit and illicit use of psychoactive drugs is difficult. Basing it on their source (medical or non-medical) is not sufficient, because obtaining a psychoactive drug from a medical source does not guarantee its therapeutic use. In the case of psychoactive drugs, a study conducted with female psychoactive drug users in three Spanish Autonomous Communities revealed that use through prescription and personal consumption, favoured by social permissiveness, is associated with the "discontent" and stress that they suffer due to the lack of models, work overload and/or emotional strain (Romo and Gil 2006). Health surveys conducted in Spain have reported that around 10% of the female population had consumed a tranquilizer without medical prescription in the previous month (Hidalgo et al. 2000). The consumption pattern for non-prescribed tranquilizers appears to be related to new modes of female drug consumption in Spain. These are legal substances when medically prescribed, but are considered illegal when their use is not under the control of a healthcare professional. The consumption of psychoactive drugs has undergone a transformation since the 1950s, becoming widespread among individuals with no psychological disease, especially females (Romo et al. 2003; Gil- García et al. 2005; Arrizaga 2007).

Some adolescent females are treated with psychoactive drugs by their physician. Others start to use them without a medical prescription, although they often obtain them from family members or friends for whom they have been prescribed (Romo et al. 2003). These self-prescribers have been described as generally healthy individuals who simultaneously begin to consume other legal and illegal drugs; in both cases (medical and self-prescription), the girls perceive the risk associated with psychoactive drugs to be low (Meneses 2002; Romo and Gil 2006).

The reasons given in the scientific literature to explain the differential use of this type of drug between men and women are varied, but there are two that my research shows as key from the point of view of gender:

- The opinion of men concerning the greater tendency of women to stress, anxiety and tension.
- Sophisticated advertisements that have defined the normative and appropriate use of these substances since the 1960s.

The reasons for this overconsumption are many, but we must bear in mind the impact of women's attention to health, and the physical and mental overload from their productive and reproductive work roles compared with men. The transformations that the family life cycle has undergone are also important, but two reasons seem the most important:

- The lower stigmatizing component that these drugs have compared to other substances.
- The low social awareness of the addictive properties of these substances.

In recent years, some groups that have broken the normativity of the heterosexual model, such as the lesbian, gay, bisexual and transgender (LGBTI) community, have begun to reflect on these addictive behaviours. It is maintained that adolescents with minority sexual orientations (lesbians, gays and bisexuals) are more likely to use drugs (illegal and prescribed) than their heterosexual peers. The differences are more accentuated during early adolescence (12–17 years old) than during later adolescence or beginnings of maturity (18–23) (Brubaker et al. 2009; Corliss et al. 2010). Other studies have shown that family support in the acceptance of their sexual identity is fundamental to the healthy behaviour of adolescents (Padilla et al. 2010; Ford and Jasinski 2006). The studies recognise that little is known about why certain differences occur or not in the use and abuse of drugs in these groups, and that further research and debate is needed on drug consumption in specific populations (Marshal et al. 2009).

5.1.2 Vulnerabilities of Gender: Gender Violence Associated with Drug Abuse and Violence Related to Drug Trafficking

The relationship of women with drugs is affected by violence in different forms. It can be viewed from different angles: the gender violence suffered at different moments of their lives when they are consumers, their involvement in the lowest and most vulnerable levels of drug trafficking, or the consumption of psychoactive substances, mostly legal, by female victims of gender violence.

In the contexts of high exclusion and vulnerability, such as those in which substances like cocaine paste are consumed in some Latin American countries, women are doubly affected by processes of stigmatization and violence (Ramírez 2015). Female consumers of substances such as cocaine paste (also known as pasta base) subvert everything that is expected of “a woman”. As a result of the survival strategies adopted in the environment in which they live, these consumers commonly participate in violent situations. They hit and are hit, rob, sell their bodies, lose contact with their families and friends and leave their children to the care of others; in other words, their actions cast doubt on the significance and practices that are attributable to “good women” (Camarotti and Touris 2010; Romo-Avilés et al. 2015).

Thus, it appears that women’s abusive consumption of substances like cocaine paste in contexts of social exclusion leads to greater possibilities of suffering situations of physical and sexual violence, not forgetting other forms of violence such as robbery or prostitution that are associated with the consumption of different drugs, setting women on trajectories that are complex, sorrowful and difficult to bear. Yet, it is likely that the ruptures that these consumers cause in the constructed and idealised model of "female identity" generate double the social rejection: they are "the other women", "poor women", and "women drug-addicts". They lose social dignity and feel the rejection of the world that surrounds them.

Currently, a key point in the debate and reflection on the impact of gender on drug dependence concerns the visibilization of women in the world of drug trafficking and their exploitation in its lowest sectors. We know that the rate of female incarceration for drug crimes has overtaken that of men. In 2012, the Open Society Foundations revealed that in the previous 5 years the female prison population in Latin America had almost doubled, from 40,000 to 74,000 inmates. The huge majority were serving sentences for minor crimes related to drug trafficking, mainly for being "mules", one of the most vulnerable links in the long drug-trafficking chain that makes millionaires of very, very few.

In all countries, more men than women (at an average of 90% of the total) entered into formal contact with the criminal justice system due to drug trafficking or possession of drugs for personal consumption. However, the presentation of data broken down according to gender has improved over the years and shows that the number of women detained for drug-related crimes has increased in absolute terms (UNODC 2016).

Once again, gender inequalities cause women's vulnerability in the face of violence, in this case because of the way in which the consequences of the illegal drug trade are suffered (Schnit zer et all, 2010). Vulnerability affects women, but also affects family members under their protection while they are in prison.

5.1.3 Gender Inequalities in the Prevention of Abuse and in the Access to Treatment for Drug Abuse

The social, psychological and biological differences between men and women condition the motivations for consuming drugs, the different patterns of use and the consequences. It istherefore essential to have a differential adaptation of the strategies directed at preventing and treating drug use and dependence in each sex. Certain aspects prove to be key for interpreting the different vulnerabilities that men and women present in the consumption of drugs (Sánchez-Pardo 2008 (Hughe s et all, 2010)). First, one must bear in mind that, despite the fact that the consumption of some substances is in general lower among women, they are more vulnerable to its effects. For example, in the case of alcohol, the threshold for risk behaviours is different in the two sexes because of differences in the metabolism of alcoholic drinks and in body weight.

Cultural, psychological and biological differences in gender demand that the strategies and activities for preventing the abusive consumption of psychoactive substances are adapted to accomodate these differences. In Latin America, the inclusion of gender perspective in drug programmes was handled in a global way, but the results have been varied and unspecific, demonstrating that there are no uniform trends in a region full of cultural, social, economical and political inequalities (Vergara and Machado 2013; Villar Márquez 2014).

In the case of preventing abusive use, a study carried out in different Latin American countries found that almost 40% of Latin American women considered that government campaigns focused on the prevention of consumption are negative or totally negative (OPDOP 2013).

The development of drug abuse prevention programmes and the treatment of addiction problems have had scant gender sensitivity. UN bodies and agencies have recognised that women face heavier burdens with regard to drug use, the health services related to drugs and when they participate in activities considered criminal according to anti-drug legislation (Open Society Foundations 2015). Women who have problems with substance abuse are frequently excluded or limited in their access to effective treatment that considers their needs and the specific circumstances of their problem (CND 2012).

One of the most interesting questions in the world of drug dependence concerns the reasons why less women reach treatment programmes than men. Part of the reason is that the programmes lack "gender perspective", which means they do not take women into account in the preparation or execution of treatment programmes, and that models and adequate intervention procedures are lacking for substance abuse by women.

In international research, the main reasons given for why drug treatment programmes are directed at men are the following:

1. Psychoactive substance abuse in women is, by preference, the consumption of legal psychoactive drugs, which do not tend to be considered a serious problem because their consequences affect the family, an area considered to be private.
2. Drug use in women generates fewer social problems than in men, who are associated with behaviours that have a greater cost for society (violence, crime, accidents, etc.).
3. Knowledge of the pharmacological action of drugs on women is more limited than for men because experimental subjects tend to be male. When women have been considered, the focus has been on the repercussions in newborn babies.
4. The research field on addictions was initially focused on the substances and, much later, on the characteristics of the users (ethnicity, age, sex, sexual orientation, etc.), with mainly white males as the model and standard of comparison, as has occurred in other fields of medicine and the health sciences.

5.2 Conclusions: Reflections on the Inclusion of Gender Perspective in Drug Dependence

Looking through the lens of gender produces a fresh view of drug dependencies; it changes some of the classic concepts, such as addiction, but above all it generates possibilities for designing drug policies that are sensitive to all users, open to the regulation of substance consumption, and offer alternatives to prohibitionism.

Including gender brings different aspects to issues in which sexual identity has not been included: analysis of the prevalence of consumption; the experience of situations of violence associated with the use, abuse and traffic of drugs; and specific treatment needs.

Perhaps what is needed is to change the context of cultural and social inequality in which substances are consumed. This would entail prioritizing the empowerment of women and any other group that is affected by inequalities resulting from their sexual identity, as regards their development in different social contexts, not only in contexts of the use and abuse of drugs.

References

Arrizaga, C. (2007). *La Medicalización de la Vida Cotidiana. El Consumo Indebido de Psicotrópicos en Adultos*. Buenos Aires: Observatorio Argentino de Drogas, SEDRONAR.

Bowleg, L. (2012). The problem with the phrase women and minorities: Intersectionality an important theoretical framework for public health. *American Journal of Public Health, 102*(7), 1267–1273.

Brubaker, M. D., Garrett, M. T., & Dew, B. J. (2009). Examining the relationship between internalized heterosexism and substance abuse among lesbian, gay, and bisexual individuals: A critical review. *Journal of LGBT Issues in Counseling, 3*(1), 62–89.

Buttler, J. (2007). *El Feminismo y la subversión de la identidad*. México: Editorial Paidós.

Calafat, A., Juan, M., Becoña, E., Mantecón, A., & Ramón, A. (2009). Sexualidad de riesgo y consumo de drogas en el contexto recreativo. Una perspectiva de género. *Psicothema, 21*(2), 227.

Camarotti, A. C., & Touris, C. (2010). Consumo/uso de pasta base en mujeres de zonas marginalizadas del sur de la Ciudad de Buenos Aires. en Artemisa. Disponible en: Retrieved from http://www.artemisanoticias.com.ar/images/FotosNotas/Mujeres%20PACO%20%20Camarotti%20Touris.pdf

CND. (2012). *Resolution 55/5. Promoting strategies and measures addressing special needs of women in the context of comprehensive and integrated drug demand reduction programmes and strategies*. Vienna, Austria: Commission on Narcotic Drugs (CND).

Connell, R. (2012). Gender, health and theory: Conceptualizing the issue, in local and world perspective. *Social Science & Medicine, 74*(11), 1675–1683.

Corliss, H. L., Rosario, M., Wypij, D., Wylie, S. A., Frazier, A. L., & Austin, S. B. (2010). Sexual orientation and drug use in a longitudinal cohort study of US adolescents. *Addictive Behaviors, 35*(5), 517–521.

Crenshaw, K. (1991). Demarginalizing the intersection of race and sex: A black feminist critique of antidiscrimination doctrine, feminist theory, and antiracist politics. En K. T. Bartlett, & R. Kennedy (Eds.), Feminist legal theory (pp. 57–80). Boulder: Westview.

DGPNSD. (2010). Encuesta Estatal sobre el Uso de Drogas en Estudiantes de Enseñanzas Secundarias (ESTUDES). España: Delegación del Gobierno para el Plan Nacional sobre Drogas (DGPNSD), Ministerio de Sanidad, Servicios sociales e Igualdad. Retrieved July 27, 2017, from http://www.pnsd.msssi.gob.es/profesionales/sistemasInformacion/sistemaInformacion/pdf/ESTUDES_2010.pdf

DGPNSD. (2016). *Encuesta Estatal sobre el Uso de Drogas en Estudiantes de Enseñanzas Secundarias (ESTUDES)*. España: Delegación del Gobierno para el Plan Nacional sobre Drogas (DGPNSD), Ministerio de Sanidad, Servicios sociales e Igualdad. Retrieved from http://www.pnsd.msssi.gob.es/profesionales/sistemasInformacion/sistemaInformacion/pdf/2016_ESTUDES_2014-2015.pdf.

Ettorre, E. (1992). *Women and substance abuse*. New Brunswick: Rutgers University Press.

Ford, J. A., & Jasinski, J. L. (2006). Sexual orientation and substance use among college students. *Addictive Behaviors, 31*(3), 404–413.

García-Calvente, M. M., Delgado, A., Mateo, I., Maroto, G. y Bolívar, J. (2008). El género como determinante de desigualdades en salud y en la utilización de servicios sanitarios en Andalucía. Primer Informe sobre Desigualdades y Salud en Andalucía, 127–143.

Gil-García, E., Avilés, N. R., Ruiz, M. P., Falcón, C. M., Alonso, I. M., & Fuente, A. V. (2005). Género y psicofármacos: la opinión de los prescriptores a través de una investigación cualitativa. *Atención primaria, 35*(8), 402–407.

Hidalgo, I., Garrido, G., & Hernández, M. (2000). Health status and risk behavior of adolescents in the north of Madrid, (Spain). *Journal of Adolescent Health, 27*(5), 351–360.

Kandall, S. R. (2010). Women and drug addiction: A historical perspective. *Journal of Addictive Diseases, 29*(2), 117–126.

Klee, H. (2001). Women, family and drugs. In H. Klee, M. Jackson, & S. Lewis (Eds.), *Drug misuse and motherhood*. London: Routledge.

Llort, A., Ferrando, S., Borrás, T. y Purroy, I. (2013). El doble estigma de la mujer consumidora de drogas: estudio cualitativo sobre un grupo de auto apoyo de mujeres con problemas de abuso de sustancias. Alternativas, Cuadernos de Trabajo Social, 20, 9–22.

Mahalingam, R., Balan, S., & Haritatos, J. (2008). Engendering immigrant psychology: An intersectionality perspective. *Sex Roles, 59*(5–6), 326–336.

Márkez Alonso, I. (2010). Dependencias: de la coerción a la reducción de daños. *Crítica, 60*(967), 33–38.

Maqueira, Virginia. (2006). Mujeres, globalización y derechos humanos 3. Cátedra. Colección feminismos.

Marshal, M. P., Friedman, M. S., Stall, R., & Thompson, A. L. (2009). Individual trajectories of substance use in lesbian, gay and bisexual youth and heterosexual youth. *Addiction, 104*(6), 974–981.

McCall, L. (2005). The complexity of intersectionality. *Signs: Journal of Woman in Culture and Society, 30*(3), 1771–1800.

Measham, F. (2002). Doing gender - doing drugs: Conceptualising the gendering of drugs cultures. *Contemporary Drug Problems, 29*(2), 335–373.

Meneses, C. (2002). De la morfina a la heroína: el consumo de drogas en las mujeres. *Miscelánea Comillas: Revista de Ciencias Humanas y Sociales, 60*(116), 217–243.

OAS and CICAD. (2011). Informe del uso de drogas en las Américas. Washington: Organization of American States (OAS) and Inter-American Drug Abuse Control Control Commission (CICAD). Retrieved from http://www.cicad.oas.org/oid/pubs/Uso_de_Drogas_en_Americas2011_Esp.pdf

OPDOP. (2013). *Segundo informe: Políticas de drogas, narcotráfico, consumo y la mujer*. Santiago: Observatorio Latinoamericano de Políticas de Drogas y Opinión Pública (OPDOP) y Asuntos del Sur (ADS). Retrieved from http://www.pensamientopenal.com.ar/system/files/2017/01/miscelaneas44694.pdf.

Open Society Foundations. (2015). *The impact of dug policy on women*. New York.

Padilla, Y. C., Crisp, C., & Rew, D. L. (2010). Parental acceptance and illegal drug use among gay, lesbian, and bisexual adolescents: Results from a national survey. *Social Work, 55*(3), 265–275.

Paechter, C., 2003. Masculinities and femininities as CoPs. *Women's Studies International Forum, 26*(1), 69–77.

Ramírez, R. (2015). Experiencias de Jóvenes ex usuarios de PB/paco en hospitales y centros de salud. En S. Sustas, S. Tapia y M. Güelman (Coord.), XI Jornadas de Sociología. Facultad de Ciencias Sociales, Buenos Aires, Argentina. Retrieved from http://jornadasdesociologia2015.sociales.uba.ar/wpcontent/uploads/ponencias/1005_334.pdf

Romo, N., Vega, A., Meneses, C., Gil, E., Márkez, I., & Poo, M. (2003). Sobre el malestar y la prescripción: un estudio sobre los usos de psicofármacos por las mujeres. *Revista Española de Drogodependencias, 28*(4), 372–380.

Romo, N. y Gil, E. (2006). Género y uso de drogas. De la ilegalidad a la legalidad para enfrentar el malestar. *Trastornos adictivos, 8*(4), 243–250.

Romo, N. (2010). La mirada de género en el abordaje de los usos y abusos de drogas. *Revista española de drogodependencias, 3*, 269–272.

Romo, N. (2011). Cannabis, juventud y género: nuevos patrones de consumo, nuevos modelos de intervención. *Trastornos adictivos, 13*(3), 91–93.

Romo, N., Meneses, C. y Gil, E. (2014). "Learning to be a girl". Gender, risks and legal drugs amongs Spanish teenagers. En T. Ortiz y M. J. Santesmases (Eds.), Gendered drugs and medicine: Historical and socio-cultural perspectives. Farnham: Ashgate.

Romo-Avilés, N., Camarotti, A. C., Tarragona, A., & Touris, C. (2015). Doing gender in a toxic world. Women and freebase cocaine in the City of Buenos Aires (Argentina). *Substance Use & Misuse, 50*(5), 557–565.

Romo-Avilés, N., Marcos-Marcos, J., Marquina-Márquez, A., & Gil-García, E. (2016). Intensive alcohol consumption by adolescents in southern Spain: The importance of friendship. *International Journal of Drug Policy, 31*, 138–146.

Romo-Avilés, N., Marcos-Marcos, J., Tarragona-Camacho, A., Gil-García, E., & Marquina-Márquez, A. (2016). "I like to be different from how I normally am": Heavy alcohol consumption among female Spanish adolescents and the unsettling of traditional gender norms. *Drugs: Education, Prevention and Policy*, 1–11.

Sánchez-Pardo, L. (2008). *Drogas y perspectiva de género. Documento marco*. Xunta de Galicia. Servizo Galego de Saúde.

SEDRONAR. (2017). *Estudio 2017 de consumo de sustancias psicoactivas*. Buenos Aires: Presidencia de la Nación. Retrieved July 27, 2017, from observatorio.gov.ar/index.php/epidemiologia/item/16-estudios-de-poblacion-general

Simien, E. M. (2007). Doing intersectionality research: From conceptual issues to practical examples. *Politics and Gender, 3*(2), 264–271.

SAMHSA. (2014). *Results from the 2013 National Survey on drug use and health: Summary of National Findings*. Rockville, MD: Substance Abuse and Mental Health Services Administration (SAMHSA).

UNODC. (2016). *World Drug Report 2016*. Brussels: United Nations Office on Drugs and Crime (UNODC).

Vergara, E., & Machado, F. (2013). *Política de drogas, narcotráfico, consumo y la mujer*. Santiago: Observatorio Latinoamericano de política de drogas y opinión pública, Asuntos del sur.

Villar Márquez, E. (2014). *Perspectiva de género y programas sobre drogas: El abordaje de las desigualdades*. Madrid: Consorcio COPOLAD.

World Health Organization. (2009). Women and health: Today's evidence tomorrow's agenda. Geneva: WHO. Disponible en: Retrieved July 27, 2017, from http://www.who.int/gender/documents/9789241563857/en/index.html

Chapter 6
Drugs and Race

Adriana Eiko Matsumoto, Marcio Farias, and Silvio Luiz de Almeida

Abstract The relationship between drugs and racism must be understood from multiple determinations in order to avoid establishing a mechanistic relationship between these two poles or drawing from overlapping contexts that do little to reveal the movements that constitute structuring elements of contemporary social reality. In this sense, the objective of this article is to demonstrate that the link between racism and the drug war is political, and depends on the performance of the State and the legal treatment given, whose logic is determined by the economy. In short, drug policy plays a fundamental role in the constitution of race as a means of power and domination; in other words, drug policy is one of the ways in which racism materializes in social life. In the first part of the article, we discuss the relationship between racism and drugs under the prism of political economy, connecting the links between the logic of materialistic reproduction of capitalist society and the mechanisms of social control. In the second part, we demonstrate how racism and the illegality of drugs are created by state intervention and manipulation of legal categories. Finally, we discuss the intersection between race and drugs and how it presents itself as a way of regulating capitalist social relations, especially in times of crisis.

A. E. Matsumoto (✉)
Department of Psychology, Universidade Federal Fluminense, Niterói, Brazil
e-mail: adrianaeiko@id.uff.br

M. Farias
Núcleo de Estudos Afro Americanos (Nepafro)/Museu Afro Brasil, São Paulo, Brazil
e-mail: t_mfarias@hotmail.com

S. L. de Almeida
Department of Political and Economic Law, Universidade Presbiteriana Mackenzie, São Paulo, Brazil
e-mail: silviovlq@gmail.com

T. M. Ronzani (ed.), *Drugs and Social Context*,
https://doi.org/10.1007/978-3-319-72446-1_6

6.1 Capitalism, Racism, and Drugs

As noted by the British sociologist Paul Gilroy (2007), the analytical sentence pronounced by W.E.B. Du Bois, "The problem of the twentieth century is the problem of the color line" (Du Bois 1999), describes a phenomenon without resolution that has carried through to the twenty-first century. Race is an antinomy (Gilroy 2001) of modernity and its roots extend to the most varied spheres of social life. The challenge of understanding race relations in the contemporary world lies in the idea that "race" is a controversial term; the relation between this term and its significance is permeated by symbolic polysemies that organize the life and sociability of groups.

As a biological attribute, there are no human races. However, in the field of social and political relations, "race" is a social conflict that accompanied the emergence of modern society. According to the anthropologist Munanga (2004), the etymology of the word "race" refers to the Latin *ratio*, which means, among other definitions, category and species. The differentiation of species used by the biological sciences was an exemplary justification for European and American intellectuals in the second half of the nineteenth century and early twentieth century. Throughout the twentieth century, with the advancement of genetic studies, it was shown that small differences between human groups do not effectively shape divisions and subdivisions between races. Thus, the idea of human race as a biological attribute falls apart.

However, what is observed in reality is that, even with the dismissal of eugenic knowledge, the idea of inferiority and superiority between races is perpetrated in the ideological field, reverberating in social relations. In this sense, nineteenth century racism is instituted in the twentieth century as "an ideological weapon of domination" (Moura 1994a). That is, racism is an ideology whose elaboration accompanies and justifies expansion of the elites of imperial and colonizing nations of the North over nations dominated or to be dominated from the South (Moore 2010).

These dominated nations, through the conformation of capitalism and objectification in their territories, have the ideology of racism as an important means of regulating asymmetrical social relations. In this way, racism is also present among the popular sectors of non-European nations and it is not only effective as a mechanical expression of the class struggle (between white bourgeoisie and black and indigenous workers), but also as an instrument of division and perpetuation of inequalities among whites, blacks, and indigenous workers (Moura 1976).

In general, white workers, whether in colonial societies or capitalist centers, are contemplated, at least symbolically, as within the world of the dominant sectors. Within the working class, white workers produce and also reproduce discriminatory actions that perpetuate privileges. There is a kind of "narcisistic covenant" (Bento 2002) between rich and poor whites, conventionally called "whiteness." Therefore, "blackness," a term used here as identity and political category, questions this hegemony and seeks affirmation of the humanity of the fraction of workers who are overexploited and symbolically demeaned, who denied and still currently deny the imposed norms, thus establishing a counter-hegemony of modernity (Gilroy 2001).

Therefore, to evoke race is not only a reverberation of a colonial past (Fernandes 2015), or a problem that was covered in its completeness by the neoliberal perspective of the twentieth century (Wood 2003), or even a problem of alterity (Balibar and Wallerstein 1991). Race is an element that constitutes the class struggle in modernity (Losurdo 2015). Evocation of race happens on the productive sphere (Rodney 1975) according to a national reality, focusing on the depreciation of the higher-value or ratifying divisions among the fractions of the working class. Moreover, the conception of race is distinguished from the productive sphere, establishing a noncausal and immediate relation to production, ultimately determined by the mode of production.

Therefore, it should be noted that racism and capitalism are intertwined. Historically, capitalism has become constituted as a racially unequal society such that, in certain national realities (in Brazil for example), the modern society of classes coexists with stratified societies. As a modern society of classes, Brazilian society, like many other countries in America, racialized in its structure, configured a stratified society for black and indigenous workers. At the same time, the white working class experienced a dynamic, competitive, but permeable society from the point of view of the oscillation of class composition, because, of course, these changes did not interfere with the structure of relations of production. Thus, it is possible to have some sort of advancement among the white working class (Ianni 1989).

On the other hand, the low social mobility in the labor market of the black and indigenous population reverberated in a kind of social ostracism for these populations. Poor access to education, housing, health, public security, social protection, and the social security system, among other aspects of bourgeois citizenship, resulted in a wide range of social vulnerabilities to which these social groups were and are subjected (Hasembalg 1979). Here, the analytic sentence of Du Bois is confirmed. Contemporary social problems in the advanced capitalist society end up being almost figures of speech for the issue of race. Furthermore, the management of these problems in competitive and antagonistic societies, in their constitutions of class and race, therefore, passes through the class struggle (Losurdo 2015).

Thus, the idea of race is operated as an ideology and, as such, accompanied and metamorphosed according to the reorganization of capital. Race is a dynamizer of the class struggle, which has become globalized according to the crises and reorganizations of the capitalist mode of production throughout the centuries. This way, the political actions conducted by agents of black activism occur in an unequal and combined way, not only orchestrated by singular challenges, but also universal. A transnational antiracist struggle was only possible because of the full and global development of capitalism, although blacks who were politically organized responded to this experience of asymmetric racialization in the aesthetic and political domains in their local, national, and continental realities.

The issue of drugs from the anti-hegemonic point of view – that is, from the black social movement throughout the twentieth and twenty-first centuries – emerged through an interface debate, which correlated the pattern of substance use by the black population with racism and its coping mechanisms. An emblematic example is from the 1969 debates of the Black Panther Party:

> Regarding black people, our problems are aggravated and assume alarming dimensions due to the racial dehumanization that we are submitted to. To understand the relationship between the plague and the black people, we must analyze the effects of capitalist exploitation and racist dehumanization ... Since the reality of our objective existence seemed to confirm the racist doctrines of white superiority and its antithesis, black inferiority, and since we failed to understand our condition, we internalized the racist propaganda of our oppressors... The misery of our suffering, our sense of helplessness, and the despair created within our minds create a pre-disposition for the use of any substance that produces euphoric illusions. We developed a complex of escapism. This escapist complex is self-destructive (Black Panther Party 2017, p. 150).

This excerpt presents the idea that the correlation between capitalism and racism has had harmful effects for black people. The processes of production, circulation, and commercialization of drugs and the racial problem were, and still are, significant obstacles to the emergence of freedom for the black population. Ultimately, the debate on race and drugs for the Black Panthers could not be dissociated from the capitalist mode of production.

In outlining counter-hegemonic movements in the relationship between drugs and race, it is essential to understand the political and analytical validity of some of the great figures of the Pan-Africanist movement, who rose and affirmed themselves in the nineteenth century and had their apex during the first half of the twentieth century (Nascimento 1981). An illustrious international case under the auspices of the international antiracist struggle, although based on local and national experiences, is the case of pan-Africanist Marcus Garvey (1887–1940) and his reflections on the Rastafari movement. The "Africa for Africans" and "Back to Africa" movements orchestrated by Garvey had a metaphorical force that enabled the action of thousands of black men and women affiliated to the Universal Negro Improvement Association (UNIA). Among these affiliates, both in the USA and the Caribbean, most black workers living in precarious conditions encountered an earthly redemption from daily hardships in the Ethiopian struggle and victory against the attempted domination intended by Italy at the end of the nineteenth century. This military and political success, under the shrewd leadership of the king, Menelick II (1844-1913), was maintained by Haile Selassie (1892-1975), whose birth name was Tafari Makonnen when he took over the Ethiopian throne in the 1930s and became "Ras," which in Amharic literally means "head" and is used to refer, in its social meaning, to princes or chiefs.

History has other fluxes and refluxes that it not possible to recount at this time – and are not the objective of this article. However, I would like to emphasize that the idea of historical belonging to another social system, different in type and degree from modern capitalist and European societies, is characteristic of this platform of militant action. Because Garvey's idea of returning to the sacred land occurred at the time of the Ras Tafari in Ethiopia, the myth had a foundation and a real bastion. Haile Selassie was the king to be worshiped and the African sacred land became Ethiopia. The modern Rastáfari religion was created then. In this worldview, the element "ganja" (marijuana) constitutes a set of practices and is the substance that has the function of spiritual explanation and elevation (Bezerra 2012). Therefore, confrontation with Eurocentric racism and the imposition of a culture that disconnected Africans and their descendants from their true origin and history had in the Rastafarians a new platform:

> Its main themes are the proclamation of Africa (and also Zion or Ethiopia) as the original cradle of humanity; the rejection of Western society (which they call Babylon, making a metaphor with the new Christian testament); the spiritual use of cannabis; peace; love; the unity; solidarity and equality among nations. Also highlighting as central themes are the repatriation of African Americans to Africa and the various social and political demands, such as Pan-Africanism, one of the claims that arose with Marcus Garvey, considered by Rastas the prophet of the movement, his correspondent in Christianity would be João Batista (Romero 2012, p. 209).

Contemporary with this expression of the American and Caribbean antiracist struggle was the Brazilian Black Front, although with other perspectives of confrontation regarding the questions of race and drugs. It was the first modern expression of the antiracist struggle carried out by blacks in Brazil, a movement that was created during the second and third decades of the twentieth century. Its predecessors were the recreational clubs and associations, which were attended by black individuals from the working class, connected to service, education, and public service sectors. They were somewhat distant from the black pauperized masses who were subjected to post-abolition plunder, because it was not possible to enter the formal labor market, often being integrated only as domestic workers. These spaces were based on the integration of the "man of color" and on the victory over the misfortunes left by slavery and retaken by racism.

The black press used newspapers to disseminate the ideas of these groups, using moralization directed at the black population, such as the incentive to marriage, orderly social life, study, and, above all, overcoming drug and alcohol addictions. This movement was the foundation of the Brazilian Black Front (Frente Negra Brasileira; FNB) regarding they way and practice of political action. Newspapers took many different approaches to the varied subjects regarding the condition of the black population and the confrontation necessary to overcome the social obstacles, using an integrationist postulate. For this reason, the relationship between the black political vanguard of this period and the whole black population was based on the idea that certain addictions, inherited from the times of slavery, should be overcome, including the use of legal and illegal substances, which socially prevented the full integration of black people into class society.

This phase of the Brazilian antiracist struggle is complex in its course; however, we focus on the more general aspects that help us understand the relationship between race and drugs, focusing on the correlation between capitalism and the antiracist struggle, without elaborating on specific elements of that period (Gomes 2005). What is pertinent to the proposed discussion are the ways in which the antiracist struggle has intersections with other complex social phenomena, in this case, drugs. The convergences and divergences of the cited cases lie in the fact that, in both cases, there is a diagnosis that racism is an obstacle and reverberates under unequal material and symbolic conditions for the black population.

In the American (the Black Panthers) and Jamaican (the Rastafari Movement) experiments, a break with capitalist modernity was the solution, in the face of other attitudes and forms of political organization that allowed a horizon of denial of the subaltern condition through a reconnection with history and senses lost as a result of colonial violence. In the Brazilian case, the modeling of attitudes as a form of integration in the society of class was the exit for Brazilian antiracist activists in the 1920s. Thus, abusive use of substances considered socially negative was a behavior to be avoided by "individuals of color," a term used by this segment at the time (Gomes 2005).

Thus, the contradictions created within these processes find permanence in the present and must be taken into account in an analysis of the phenomenon of drugs and racism based on the totality of concrete social relations, focusing mainly on the production, movement, and consumption of illicit substances.

6.2 State and Law: The Structural Links between Race and Drugs

Given the elements presented, and in order to broaden our understanding of the foundations of the relationship between race and drugs, it is necessary to analyze conceptions of the State and the law regarding their connection with capitalism. We start from the idea that the State and the law not only function as external connectors between the racial problem and the drug policy, but above all as elements that manifest a *structural link* between them. In other words, both the racial issue and the drug problem, as manifested in contemporary social relations, are *internally* and *externally* linked to the State and the law, which makes it possible the problems of race and drugs are linked to the performance of the State and the categorizations engendered by law. In the same way, observing the relationship between racial politics and drug policy allows us to capture how the State and the law express themselves within capitalist society.

Far from idealist and/or legal positivist conceptions of the State as a "common good," the "synthesis of the interests of civil society," or a "set of rules" and also far from the supposedly realistic view recognizing the State only as a mere "apparatus of power of the bourgeoisie" or "real factor of power," the State is here defined as the expression of the structural conditions of an economically organized society based on private production, wage labor, and commodity exchange (Hirsch 2010; Mascaro 2013; Caldas 2015). In a society with such characteristics, political power is not expressed as the direct domination of a class or certain groups, but in the form of a centralized power that mediates between free, equal, and proprietary individuals. In this case, "exercising mediation" means keeping a society under a control that acts for antagonistic and even contradictory interests, through the systematic use of violence or the production of a social imagine that "normalizes" conflicts and "naturalizes" the places that each individual "occupies" in society.

Like the State, the law is a social form like any other, and is determined by the capitalist system. In this sense, the law materializes as a relationship among legal *subjects*, that is, among free and equal individuals who are in the position of being owners. Thus, the *subject form (legal form)* is a consequence of the *mercantile form* (Marx, 2014; Pachukanis, 2017).

The condition of legal subject allows all necessary social work to be reduced to abstract work.

> It is only with the full development of bourgeois relations that the law assumed an abstract character. Every man becomes a man in general, every job becomes work in general, each individual becomes an abstract legal subject. At the same time norm assumes, equally, the logical form of the abstract general law (Pachukanis, 2017).

Law is not just an ideology. Law is *also* an ideology, in the sense that it is necessary for individuals to introduce the naturalness of their free and equal condition. For this to happen, the existence of a state judicial apparatus is fundamental. We call this apparatus, with an ideological accent, a *justice system*. It can, paradoxically, guarantee liberty and equality through force, as well as guard over property, in cases where the psychological mechanisms of the individual and the inculcation of capitalist ethico-moral standards are not sufficient for social conditions to be internalized.

The legal relation gains shape when the necessary equivalence is established, not only among goods (objects), but also among those who exchange the goods (subjects). After all, a contract, including labor contracts, can only be made between free and equal people, a condition that is only established as necessary to the economic process in capitalism when labor must be predominantly free. It is worth noting that the same logic of equivalence and free will is embedded in criminal law. Penalties apply only to those who practice certain conduct by "free and conscious will," the same autonomy of will of the subject of the contract, whose meaning remains in the exchange. In general, an attempt is made to establish an equivalence, a form of "rationality" in deciding punishment, which supposedly depends on the "seriousness" of the act practiced. As a rule (except in cases where the expected punishment is death), the punishment is the result of an exchange of the conduct practiced by the individual by his free time or his money (in the case of a fine). It is not by chance that the ideological conceptions of criminal law maintain that criminals break the "social contract"; thus, legal subjectivity is the starting point of law as a social relation, no matter which "area" of law.

The law presupposes a relationship among legal subjects. It was because of the absence of autonomy of will that slaves in the USA and Brazil until the nineteenth century, as well as in the French and English colonies, were not considered legal subjects, but legal objects (property) or, at most, "crime subjects." This view explains the treatment of the enslaved as "things" under private law, but as defendants in criminal law, with different (stiffer) penalties for the same conduct because of their slave condition. Hence, mass incarceration, the drug war, and racism can only be partially treated as a legal problem, because criminalization involves the classification of individuals as legal subjects. The laws aims to eliminate the historical conditions under which practices considered criminal, such as drug trafficking, come into being. However, the law is not able to provide a reasonable explanation as to why drug criminalization has particularly dire effects on the black population.

The practices that constitute capitalism are marked by acts that are often not provided by law or are even expressly prohibited by law. The enormous amounts of money trafficked annually within the financial system are proof that capitalism is not reproduced solely by legality (Pachukanis, 2017; Mascaro 2013). What may or may not be "private property" and, consequently, an object of contract between legal subjects is a political and economic decision, that, eventually, gains legal contours. Hence, it can be concluded that the "lawfulness" and "unlawfulness" of the use of a substance become the content of a norm as a result of political and economic criteria.

It is through an analysis of political economy that capitalism, racism, and state control of drugs begins to be delineated. To do so, we return to conflict as a structural category of capitalism. The conflict between capital and wage labor is not the only conflict in capitalist society. There are other conflicts that are articulated by the relations of domination and exploitation, which do not originate in class relations or "disappear with it" (Hirsch 2010, p. 86): They are racial, sexual, religious, cultural, and regional conflicts that take a specifically capitalist form. The relationship between the State and society is not limited to the exchange and production of commodities. Relations of oppression of sexual and racial exploitation are important in defining the mode of state intervention and in organizing the general aspects of society; this points to a *structural nexus* between class relations and the social constitution of racial and sexual groups.

We can conclude that, in a society structurally divided by virtue of its economic logic, the State is the main factor of integration, either through institutionalized violence or through support of the image of nationality, in which cultural and ideological ties between individuals are built. Such ties are attributed to a common language, religion, cultural habits, or physical characteristics, which many synthesize in the race category.

In countries such as Brazil, the USA, and South Africa, racism is not a factor of social disintegration or even hindrance to the formation of a national identity. On the contrary, the history of these countries shows that the constitution of their respective economies and the production of a national identity were made through racialization, more precisely with the systematic discrimination of Africans and their descendants. The social and economic histories of Brazil, the USA, and South Africa cannot be properly told without an analysis of the decisive role of the State in slavery, apartheid, and, currently, in the drug war, whose boundaries are undeniable racial (Alexander 2010).

In capitalism, political relations take the form of a State that is impersonal and external to social life but, paradoxically, "stabilizes" society by maintaining the processes of individualization and class separation that characterize capitalism. Therefore, state control of society takes place through the legal classification of individuals, so that their subjective identities are directly related to the process of social reproduction. By the action of the State and normative conformation operated by the law, individuals are the subjects of rights, citizens, voters, and employees, but are also racialized subjects who are socially and economically positioned according to the racial group to which they belong.

The topic of territory in the relation between race, drugs, State, and law also deserves attention. It is essential for the social control that the State is able to make territorial plans and, with this, effect the control and surveillance of the population. Territorial demarcation is central to the process of classifying people and, consequently, adapting subjectivities to social life (Foucault 2004). Birth control, definition of the criteria of entry and permanence in the territory according to elements of nationality determined by law, creation of *ghettos* or reserves for certain social groups, legal recognition of territories or collective properties according to the identity of the group (*quilombolas*, indigenous people, etc.), and even imprisonment are all examples of how the State cannot be conceived without territoriality. Indeed, racialization is the result of an identity-space policy. Blacks and whites occupy different places in the territorial space, which is reflected in the logic of public security policies and in police interventions in the peripheral areas, where the vast majority are nonwhite. This same territoriality articulated by the State makes sense for the "territories of trafficking," which are generally where a large proportion of the poor and the black live. These territories are also where the expression "drug war" becomes literal, using weapons and military apparatus, which would not be admitted in the neighborhoods and localities of white and middle-class residents.

Thus, reflecting on race and drugs from the perspective presented here means to articulate the analyzed elements (capitalist mode of production, racism, the State, and law) in their relation with the totality.

6.3 The War on Drugs as an Expression of Racism in the Era of Capital Crisis

In order to discuss the "War on Drugs" in its racialized constitution and class perspective, it is crucial to understand the current movement that constitutes the state-form, as well as the segmentations in law and the relations between drugs and race.

We believe that it is important to consider the dynamics of the crisis in capitalism, because to define it is to determine, to some extent, the functioning not only of the economy, but also of political institutions that must maintain stability and that relate to the State (Hirsch 2010, p. 134). The process of capitalist production depends on permanent expansion of production and incessant accumulation of capital. However, these factors find historical limits that clash with the conflicting characteristics of society. Crisis is expressed when the processes of the capitalist economy are not compatible with the institutions and norms that should maintain stability. Thus, crises reveal the inability of the capitalist system at certain moments in history to promote social integration through the existing social rules. In other words, the mode of regulation, as constituted by legal norms, values, and mechanisms of institutional conciliation and integration, conflicts with the regime of accumulation (Aglietta 2000). The consequence is that the link between the State and civil society, maintained through the use of repressive and ideological mechanisms, reaches its limit. The regulatory system collapses, resulting in conflicts between state institutions, independence from government agencies that turn against each other, lack of government direction, and political instability.

Crises, therefore, challenge new forms of state intervention in order to establish modes of social control that can continue capitalist accumulation within some regularity. Historically, the great crises of capitalism have resulted in different strategies of state intervention in order to adapt society to the demands of capitalist production, which have had a profound impact on racial politics. It is possible, within such a perspective, to tell a history of the crises of capitalism that parallels the history of contemporary racism. The first great crisis of 1873 resulted in imperialism and European colonialism, whose ideological bearing was the allegedly "scientific" racism against Africa, Latin America, and Asia. The Great Depression of 1929 resulted in social welfare policies and the integration of social groups into the labor market and consumption, which did not mean the end of racism because people belonging to racial and cultural minorities were paid less and had precarious living conditions. This situation was illustrated by the interaction of the welfare state and the Fordist regime of accumulation in the USA, which led to racial segregation in the South until the 1960s. The relationship between the process of industrialization and the emergence of the ideology of racial democracy in Brazil still serves to prevent recognition of the political and economic inequality between whites and blacks.

The current crisis of the Fordist model and the welfare state has its most evident effects in the extermination and imprisonment of the poor and black populations who, under neoliberal economics, are cut off from the consumer market and have the product of their work turned to financial returns. In this last facet of the attempt at neoliberal regulation, the war on drugs introduces a "new Jim Crow," as named by Michelle Alexander (2010).

In fact, since the mid-1990s, there has been a worldwide trend of increasing incarceration rates. Although there are specific characteristics in each continent, country, and culture, a hegemonic way of criminalizing and arresting is present in most parts of the world. The articulation between repressive policies and the class issues are derived from structural racism and xenophobic actions that are part of this panorama.

Thus, in view of the contributions of critics of the political economy, we are interested in analyzing the processes that are in the midst of the constitution of the drug war by taking the drug as a commodity made illicitly but produced, distributed and consumed in different ways.

In 1971, US president Richard Nixon publicly declared a War on Drugs that later spread throughout the world. The "dangerousness" preached as a fundamental characteristic of the production, trade, and consumption of illicit substances had to be faced with drastic and oppressive measures (Rodrigues 2004). We can see in this process the legitimacy, increasingly potentiated, of state intervention in relative individual freedoms, under the prohibitionist paradigm.

Therefore, there is no way to understand the complex relations of the drug war without outlining how the production processes of mass entrapment are structured, taking into consideration those countries that have higher incarceration rates and are in economic dependency (combined and uneven) with the countries of central capitalism, with special attention to the countries of Latin America, and notably Brazil.

This configuration is determined by multiple elements, such as the processes of overexploitation of work, which is typical of neoliberalist politics in times of a structural crisis of capital, and reordering of the legal and legislative spheres under the aegis of zero tolerance. In any case, criminal selectivity operates, in these and other countries, from the configuration of state racism. The project of mass incarceration is a tributary of the relations set by the State in its racist constitution and social control, with a widespread use of institutional violence toward the working class, which finds social justification for implementation in the drug war.

According to the report "Prison: Evidence of its use and over-use from around the world," there are currently 10 million people imprisoned worldwide (Jacobson et al. 2017). However, depending on the country and the phenotypic and cultural characteristics of the individual, there are greater or lesser chances of being incarcerated. It is worth noting that the USA currently has about one-fifth of the world's prison population, and Brazil has increased its contingent of incarcerated people by 20 times since 1980.

When we look at the penitentiary statistics in Brazil, regarding the profile of criminalized and imprisoned people, we observe a specific outline of the "criminal subject." These are young black men with low education, in custody and sentenced for the crime of "drug trafficking." In Latin America, regular use of the preventive detention order is common, which characterizes a specific way of mass incarceration (according to the report on the use of preventive detention in the Americas by the Inter-American Commission on Human Rights, CIDH, in 2013).

Police lethality and war operations and conflicts within and between national territories, based on the logic of combating drugs, also have effects on the militarized control of Latin American countries. Among the countries of the American continent, we highlight the process of extermination carried out by the military police in different Brazilian states.

The drug war is an effective way to criminalize the survival strategies of a large part of the population who experience daily precarious conditions. However, as we have seen, these procedures have a different effect on the subjects, because the State, since the capital crisis, has applied ostensible and repressive actions in a racialized perspective.

Thus, we can understand that the drug war is a successful example of predatory business that promotes and disseminates a sense of insecurity, which also contributes to the discrimination of new contours, a new "internal enemy," increasingly outlined in Latin American contexts, for example, in the image of black and indigenous youths. Intensification of the effective subjugation power over the popular classes is underway, developed from the control of crime that operates by the logic of racialization and consolidated by disruption of the coping possibilities of the working class against the capital. In this sense, when analyzing the drug war, we find an important axis that contributes to the reflection about the State's actions in times of capital crisis, characterized as political, economic, and social management of misery in its specificities.

References

Aglietta, M. (2000). *A theory of capitalist regulation: The US experience*. London: Verso.

Alexander, M. (2010). *The new Jim Crow: Mass incarceration in the age of colorblindness*. New York: New Press.

Balibar, É., & Wallerstein, I. (1991). *Race, nation, class: Ambiguous identities*. London: Verso.

Bento, M. A. S. (2002). *Psicologia social do racismo*. Petrópolis, RJ: Vozes.

Bezerra, D. A. P. (2012). *O movimento rastafari: da Jamaica para identidade e cultura em Fortaleza*. PhD thesis., Faculdade de Educação, Universidade Federal do Ceará, Fortaleza, CE. Retrieved from http://www.repositorio.ufc.br/handle/riufc/7602

Black Panther Party. (2017). *Todo poder ao povo: Artigos, discursos e documentos do Partido dos Panteras Negras*. São Paulo, SP: Raízes da América.

Caldas, C. (2015). *Teoria da derivação do estado e do direito*. São Paulo, SP: Dobra/Expressão Popular.

Du Bois, W. E. B. (1999). *As almas da gente negra (Gomes, H. T., trad.)*. Rio de Janeiro, RJ: Lacerda Editores.

Fernandes, F. (2015). *Poder e contra poder na América Latina*. São Paulo, SP: Expressão Popular.

Foucault, M. (2004). *Segurança, território, população*. São Paulo, SP: Martins Fontes.

Gilroy, P. (2007). *Entre campos: nações, cultura e fascínios da raça*. São Paulo: Annablume.

Gilroy, P. (2001). *O Atlântico Negro: Modernidade e dupla consciência*. São Paulo, SP/Rio de Janeiro, RJ: 34/Universidade Cândido Mendes – Centro de Estudos Afro-Asiáticos.

Goldberg, D. (2001). *The racial state*. New Jersey: Wiley-Blackwell.

Gomes, F. (2005). *Negros e política (1888–1937)*. Rio de Janeiro, RJ: Jorge Jahar.

Hasembalg, C. (1979). *Discriminação e desigualdades raciais no Brasil*. Rio de Janeiro, RJ: Graal.

Hirsch, J. (2010). *Teoria materialista do estado*. Rio de Janeiro, RJ: Renovar.

IACHR (2013) Report on the use of pretrial detention in the Americas. Inter-American Commission on Human Rights (IACHR), Organization of American Sates (OAS), Washington D.C. Available at http://www.oas.org/en/iachr/pdl/reports/pdfs/Report-PD-2013-en.pdf

Ianni, O. (1989). *Estado e capitalismo: estrutura social e industrialização no Brasil*. São Paulo, SP: Brasiliense.

Jacobson, J., Heard, C., & Fair, H. (2017). *Prison: Evidence of its use and over-use from around the world. Institute for Criminal Policy Research*. London, England: Institute for Criminal Policy Research/Fair Trials.

Losurdo, D. (2015). *A luta de classes: uma história política e filosófica*. São Paulo, SP: Boitempo.

Mascaro, A. (2013). *Estado e forma política*. São Paulo, SP: Boitempo.

Moore, C. (2010). *A África que incomoda: sobre a problematização do legado africano no quotidiano brasileiro*. Belo Horizonte, MG: Nandyala.

Moura, C. (1994a). O racismo como arma de dominação. *Revista Princípios, 34*, 28–38.

Moura, C. (1994b). *Dialética radical do Brasil negro*. São Paulo, SP: Anita.

Moura, C. (1976). *O preconceito de cor na literatura de cordel*. São Paulo, SP: Resenha Universitária.

Munanga, K. (2004). Uma abordagem conceitual das noções de raça, racismo, identidade e etnia. *Cadernos PENESB – Programa de Educação sobre o negro na sociedade brasileira, 5*, 15–34.

Nascimento, E. L. (1981). *Pan-Africanismo na América do Sul: emergência de uma rebelião negra*. São Paulo, SP: Vozes.

Rodney, W. (1975). *Como a Europa subdesenvolveu a África?* Lisboa, Portugal: Seara Nova.

Rodrigues, T. (2004). *Política e drogas nas Américas*. São Paulo, SP: EDUC/FAPESP.

Romero, Z. M. (2012). Haile Selassie I: Um deus negro ou um imperador absolutista? In: *XIII Encontro Estadual de História ANPUH-PR: A Escrita da História, 10*, Universidade Estadual de Londrina. Retrieved from https://www.academia.edu/3852760/HAILE_SELASSIE_I_UM_DEUS_NEGRO_OU_UM_IMPERADOR_ABSOLUTISTA?auto=download

Wood, E. M. (2003). *Democracia contra o capitalismo: a renovação do materialismo histórico*. São Paulo, SP: Boitempo.

Chapter 7
(Des)Occupation of Urban and Rural Spaces, Gentrification and Drug Use

Magda Dimenstein, Marcelo Dalla Vecchia, João Paulo Macedo, and Francisco Inacio Bastos

Abstract From a public policy point of view, Brazil has shown deep unhelpfulness, together with criminalization and pathologization of certain social groups and individuals, when it comes to delivering treatment to alcoholics, crack users, and others who make harmful/dependent use of substances. In 2011, with the approval of Ordinance 3.088, which instituted the Network of Psychosocial Care, there was special attention to the structure and implementation of new services such as CAPSad (Center for Psychosocial Care: Alcohol and Drugs) and the organization of care from the perspective of integrated and regionalized health networks. However, there are many weak links in this process: lack of funding, poor administration, insufficient service offer, increased competition of the private sector with public resources, lack of commitment to the principles of the SUS (Brazil's Unified Health System), weak professional training for SUS workers, cultural opposition to integration between services and professionals, power struggles in municipalities, and predominance of the instrumental-technical mindset. This chapter aims to discuss two aspects that characterize the hegemonic policy on alcohol and other drugs, as applied to the concrete case of Brazil's most deprived regions and populations: (1) Policies do not affect populations and territories in the same way, but have been particularly inadequate for social realities where people are vulnerable or socially excluded. (2) There is a very diverse reality experienced by populations who live in rural and urban regions, which has yet to be properly addressed.

M. Dimenstein (✉)
Universidade Federal do Rio Grande do Norte/UFRN, Natal, Rio Grande do Norte, Brazil
e-mail: mgdimenstein@gmail.com

M. D. Vecchia
Universidade Federal de São João Del Rei/UFSJ, São João Del Rei, Minas Gerais, Brazil
e-mail: mdvecchia@ufsj.edu.br

J. P. Macedo
Universidade Federal do Piauí/UFPI, Parnaíba, Piauí, Brazil
e-mail: jampamacedo@gmail.com

F. I. Bastos
Fundação Oswaldo Cruz/FIOCRUZ, Rio de Janeiro, Brazil
e-mail: francisco.inacio@icict.fiocruz.br

T. M. Ronzani (ed.), *Drugs and Social Context*,
https://doi.org/10.1007/978-3-319-72446-1_7

7.1 Introduction

From a public policy point of view, Brazil has shown deep unhelpfulness, together with criminalization and pathologization of certain social groups and individuals, when it comes to helping alcoholics, crack users, and others who make harmful/dependent use of substances. Until very recently, a prohibitionist ideology and an exclusive belief in abstinence as the only acceptable treatment goal were the main references of the Brazilian state on the issue of substance use in the country. It was only in 2001, with the advent of Law 10.216 (Lei da Reforma Psiquiátrica Brasileira) [Brazilian Psychiatric Reform Law] allied with the directives and policies approved by the III Conferência Nacional de Saúde Mental [III National Mental Health Conference], that it became possible to propose a new model of care, according to the harm reduction philosophy, for people with special needs as a result of harmful/dependent substance use. Thereby, a new policy of comprehensive care for users of alcohol and other substances was launched by the Brazilian Ministry of Health in 2003, characterized by the intention to guarantee universal access to comprehensive management and care for users and their families (Brazilian Ministry of Health 2003).

It was under this context that the Centro de Atenção Psicossocial em Álcool e Drogas (CAPSad) [Center for Psychosocial Care: Alcohol and Drugs] was created. CAPSad are specialized, open and community-based services, based on the principles of the Sistema Único de Saúde (SUS) [Brazil's Unified Health System], inspired by the perspectives of harm reduction and psychosocial care, that favor continuous health management and care of people with special needs resulting from the use of psychoactive substances (Brasil 2003). Because of the nature of the service and because care targets users of alcohol and other substances, CAPSad became, historically, a central facility in the network of services and facilities, as a reference point and a "gateway" for these needs and demands. For many years, CAPSad was forced to act in isolation and, therefore, became overloaded (sometimes to the point of being unable to work at all) in carrying out its institutional mission. This affected the service in terms of its capacity to enroll new patients and to highlight comprehensive clinical care, rehabilitation, and psychosocial reintegration. Its ability to help organize the local network of services, including supervising and building matrix-based activities on mental health, also became limited.

In 2011, with the approval of Ordinance 3.088, which instituted the Rede de Atenção Psicossocial (RAPS) [Network for Psychosocial Care] and established criteria for organization and implementation on mental health issues throughout the country (Brazilian Ministry of Health 2011a). Specifically, the "Policy of Care to People who Make Harmful/Dependent Use of Alcohol and other Substances" gave special attention to the structure and implementation of new services such as CAPSad and to the organization of care from the perspective of integrated and regionalized health networks. RAPS is based on the paradigm of psychosocial care and on the principles of autonomy, respect for human rights, and the exercise of citizenship. It seeks to promote equality and to recognize the social determinants of the health–illness–suffering–care process, aiming to minimize stigma and prejudices.

Its goal is to assure access to quality care, organize network services with the creation of intersectoral actions, foster continuity of care, develop actions with a territorial and communitary base, and develop permanent educational actions, as well as monitor and evaluate the effectiveness of services (Brasil 2011a).

Roughly speaking, the RAPS aims and policies are similar to the proposals for territorialization, referral and counter-referral, and integration of management and case that are present in other mental health care services worldwide, such as the French tradition of organizing different social and health care services and defense of rights by geographic zones and previously established sociodemographic selections, which is usually called "arrondissement" assistance (available, for example, in the excellent and informative online material of the care centers and crisis management facilities/services).

On organizational terms, RAPS incorporates the following different access points, facilities, and processes within the scope of SUS: (a) primary care, (b) psychosocial care, (c) urgent and emergency care, (d) residential care of transitional character, (e) hospital care, (f) deinstitutionalization strategies, and (g) psychosocial rehabilitation. The expansion of access points and a bigger diversity of services has greatly widened the coverage of services aimed at people with special needs because of their harmful/dependent use of alcohol and other substances, with a recent emphasis on extending care to small and medium-sized municipalities, the growing participation in primary care, CAPS networking (particularly between regular CAPSad and 24/7 CAPSad), and decentralization of psychosocial care beds and residential therapy services.

Despite all the efforts, including those to regionalize mental health care in the country and reach the smaller municipalities and populations living in rural and peri-urban contexts, we are far from overcoming the panorama of inequality regarding services offered and actual networking. Assistential gaps remain, especially in certain regions/localities, which means there are places in which the offer in terms of basic infrastructure and/or human resources is still insufficient or even completely absent, in clear opposition to the standards advised by public health policy to ensure psychosocial care actions, including care in cases concerning alcohol and substance use. This is the situation, for example, faced by specialized services and some of the primary health care teams as a result of important regional differences. We discuss this in further detail in Sect. 2, based on a study called "Regionalizing Alcohol and Drug Use Care in Brazil" coordinated by two authors of this chapter (Macedo et al. 2017).

In the case of hospital-based care, which is an important network point for providing care to acute cases associated with harmful/dependent substance use, in breaking-point crisis, and/or in the management of abstinence syndromes, the country only has 997 beds classified under the label "psychosocial" (as opposed to traditional, long-term psychiatric hospitalization). These beds are clustered in 193 municipalities, representing about 3.5% of the 5500 municipalities in the whole country. There are many challenges to implementation of the psychosocial beds in Brazil, such as financing and the resistance by administrators and workers due to the pervasive asylum culture and stigma that function as hurdles to the way that patients should be seen and cared for.

There are only 38 units that offer temporary residential care for people with specific needs related to use of alcohol, crack cocaine, and other substances; these people require specialized professional help and a safe place to stay for a limited period of time.

Therapeutic communities (TCs) are also elements of the RAPS and aim to provide residential care of transitory character, but instead offer long-term inpatient care and follow principles that differ from those inspired by harm reduction, psychiatric reform, and anti-asylum movements and regulations. TCs are usually guided by the philosophy of abstinence as the only acceptable treatment alternative for substance users, under the guidance of a religious/moral perspective (Bolonheis-Ramos and Boarini 2015). The inclusion of TCs in the context of RAPS has generated tension and discontentment among users, family members, and mental health workers. There are, overall, 1863 registered TCs (besides an unknown number of informal/non-registered units) across the country. The funding for TCs is provided via dedicated bids by the Secretaria Nacional de Políticas sobre Drogas (SENAD) [National Drug Policy Secretariat], part of the Ministry of Justice.

There are currently 315 CAPSad and 88 24/7 CAPSad units. Although there has been an expansion in the network regarding specialized psychosocial care, as the number of municipalities with a CAPSad service has reached 268, only 68 have 24/7 CAPs. There are still a significant number of municipalities that cannot rely on these services even though they meet the criteria for their implementation. About 214 places (50.6%) do not have access to CAPSad and 140 (79.1%) do not have access to 24/7 CAPSad. Even worse, 183 municipalities do not have access to either service (Macedo et al. 2017).

Primary care in regards to RAPS includes four components, comprising 332,289 Agentes Comunitários de Saúde [Health Community Agents], 48,410 Equipes de Saúde da Família [Family Health Teams], 5067 Núcleos de Apoio à Saúde da Família [Centers providing Support to Family Health Teams] and 135 Equipes de Consultório na Rua (CR) [Street Office Teams].

The CR teams are composed of community outreach workers who provide full care to the homeless, 52.6% of which operate in southeastern Brazil, where the largest number of homeless people live, mainly in the capitals, their impoverished outskirts, and medium-sized municipalities (Macedo et al. 2017).

The global initiative implemented by the World Health Organization prioritizes the role of primary care in mental health for a number of reasons, as detailed in their documents. One of the most important reasons is the fact that the large majority of countries do not have a large number of specialized professionals with proper training, which greatly overloads the few services and professionals with a background/focus on mental health (among a large number of publications, we would like to mention the article by Saraceno et al. 2007). The lack of facilities is a central problem in all low and average income countries such as Brazil, where the program "Mais Médicos" [More Doctors] made clear that a large number of the 5500 Brazilian municipalities do not even have a single general practitioner (GP), let alone professionals with different specialties (see the ongoing debate in the blog of the academic journal *História, Ciências, Saúde – Manguinhos*) (História, Ciências, Saúde – Manguinhos 2013).

Primary care is one of the points of the network in which it is necessary to invest in permanent educational action, as well as matrix-based mental health, on a continuous basis, with the aim of deinstitutionalizing practices and knowledge. Most of all, the aim is to curb the spread of a culture of fear and prejudice that has misguided professionals who work with people who make harmful/dependent use of substances, which, from a sociological perspective, makes them people marginalized from "normal" society, as discussed in the seminal studies by Becker (1997).

Historically, the services of primary care have been very reticent to offer mental health actions in their territories. Silveira (2009) highlights that the lack of training by professionals and lack of help for families and communities dealing with the psychic suffering and other effects caused by harmful/dependent substance use have become more evident over time. Tavares et al. (2013) conclude that health professionals are unprepared to respond to these demands, and that the difficulties in access and care for those who are suffering in the context of primary care have different underlying causes, including lack of understanding of different cultural codes when it comes to express pain and suffering; lack of proper training; the predominance of services and professionals that are still anchored in a fragmented care model; prioritizing a mental health policy for people with conditions that are considered urgent; and absence of technology that can foster care and access for patients with "fuzzy" complaints, such as vague body symptoms. The last challenge was insightfully debated by the anthropologist Luiz Fernando Duarte, in his classic work (Duarte 1986).

Sadly, in Brazil, there are still treatment regimens based on the compulsory institutionalization of patients, based exclusively on the obsessive pursuit of abstinence at all costs. This type of treatment mostly takes place in institutions that, according to Ervin Goffman's typology, are defined as "total institutions" (Goffman 1961). Interventions are provided in different combinations, but are almost invariably disharmonic and unilateral. Treatments center on medical-pharmaceutical interventions with religious overtones, leaving the user with no alternative but to "choose" between asylums, therapeutic communities, and penitentiaries. Therefore, the only alternatives left are those that render substance users as mad, degenerate, or immoral persons who should be dealt with as delinquents or criminals (Rosenstock and Neves 2010).

There are many challenges facing the teams of family health professionals under this perspective. They must work under a conceptual framework (highly prescriptive and centered on illness) that is different from that learned during their academic career; deal with their own anxieties, insecurities, and prejudices; and cope with their own inability to provide care and management to people who use alcohol and other substances. There is also a mismatch between their daily activities and the policies issued by the highest public service spheres (such as the Ministry of Health), which are not consolidated in the region and not given their proper value by local administrators. Professional must also develop protocols that allow for the monitoring and evaluation of actions targeting people who use alcohol and other substances; and, last but not least, work in a multidisciplinary team aiming to foster the comprehensive character of care (Gonçalves 2002).

Such challenges are aggravated in settings where psychosocial care delivered to people who use alcohol and other substances is restricted to primary care teams, as is the case in at least 3006 municipalities (about 54% of Brazilian municipalities), further jeopardizing access and proper response to the demands of alcohol and other substance users and their families (Macedo et al. 2017).

Of the 5607 Núcleos de Apoio à Saúde da Família (NASF) [Family Support Hubs] teams all over the country at the moment, many are located in small towns. This is an excellent indicator, considering that 54% of Brazilian municipalities only have primary care teams working with users of alcohol and other substances. On the other hand, 1798 municipalities do not have any kind of NASF, a condition that makes the RAPS even more fragile in small municipalities (Macedo et al. 2017).

To go deeper into the debate on how psychosocial care has been implemented with regards to primary care, we used data from the Programa Nacional de Melhoria do Acesso e da Qualidade da Atenção Básica (PMAQ) [National Program for Improvement of Basic Care Access] to create an analytic framework that may help in spreading this policy to the three government spheres (federal, state, and municipal), and also guarantee the administration of optimal care by the health teams, aiming to foster increased access and better quality of treatment that focuses on users' needs and satisfaction. PMAQ is inserted into the sphere of structural actions by the Ministry of Health, which focuses on primary care in an attempt to improve and assess the capacity of response to the health needs of the population.

To aid understanding of our conceptual framework, we list the key attributes that characterize primary care, as based on Starfield (2002): (a) primary care provides first contact with the (potential) clientele, (b) longitudinality, (c) comprehensiveness and integrality, and (d) coordination of care.

For the sake of the present text, the PMAQ data were analyzed to highlight the actions related to mental health and psychosocial care. The findings were initially encouraging, considering that 80.1% of teams reported implementing the program. However, 57.8% of the teams did not have qualified professionals to evaluate and properly assess the user's risk and vulnerability.

In a different context, the management and care of American heroin users with methadone, a process called "interim management and treatment," has proven to be extremely useful, with excellent results. It is especially relevant for services that often deal with overcrowding and long waiting lines (Yancovitz et al. 1991; Friedman et al. 1994).

For over a third (38.5%) of teams in Brazil, all users that arrive at the health units are immediately treated and have their needs heard and assessed. The data is bleaker regarding the spontaneous demand involving mental health cases: only 30% of teams said they did took cases in, whereas 62.0% did not know how to answer the question or did not answer anything. In regions plagued by the so-called assistance gaps, the proportion of services that did not offer the clientele the alternative of staying for a short period as inpatients was 26.1%, whereas 70.7% of the interviewees did not know or did not answer.

With respect to the interrelationship between mental health and the primary care network, the findings were not auspicious. Only 40 (i.e., 5%) of the teams in the country answered that they benefited from specific appointments in the context of a more flexible timeframe; 42.7% of teams collected the life history of their clients; and 26.4% offered some kind of group therapy. However, 66.2% of teams had not prepared their staff to deal with users with mental illnesses (dual diagnosis).

In regions with assistential gaps in their respective RAPS, the results were even worse: only 21.7% of the interviewees used specific appointments with a more flexible timeframe, 24.8% collected life histories, 11.5% offered some kind of group therapy, and 72.6% of teams did not have any proper training and lacked expertise in the management and care of users with mental illness.

Such findings compromise the ability of primary care to properly handle mental health cases and narrow their scope. The results expose an uneven offer of care, as most of the Estratégia de Saúde da Família (ESF) [Strategy for Family Health] teams in the country (58.4%) answered that they did not register the absolute number or proportion of mentally ill users in their catchment area.

Regarding cases defined as complex, 88.5% of teams answered that they benefitted from matrix-based actions (i.e., those integrating individual care and community mobilization). However, although such integration constitutes a strategy considered essential for guiding mental health operations in the context of basic care, 51.2% of researched teams did not have meetings to train teams clinically about how to better integrate their efforts with matrix-based participation (NASF, CAPS, specialized groups). On locations considered plagued by assistential gaps, this proportion increased to 67.5%. This is a matter of concern, especially because of the modest role of psychosocial care as an integral part of a primary care teams' actions (especially when they are considered in the context of [frustrated] policies and expectations). On the other hand, the uneven support offered by the teams might indicate that the matrix-based actions have not advanced, in terms of technical and pedagogical support, in their putative role of strengthening interpersonal bonds and institutional backing, in the sense of consolidating them as a key strategy for educating the clientele on a permanent basis, thus gaining firm ground to anchor therapeutic projects for disenfranchised populations (Chiaverni 2011).

The findings about the role of the psychosocial care network as a key (at least, hypothetically) component of the Brazilian Health Regionalization Policy document a worrying picture, despite advances in expanding and improving the quality of the service network and previous experience of management and care practices that correspond to the needs of drug users. Brazil is one of the few countries in the world that has a public health system based on territorial and community perspectives. Furthermore, it is one that believes in primary care as a structural axis of the system's organization and in harm reduction as a public policy, unlike hegemonic tendencies that tend to focus on abstinence as an exclusive treatment goal and on pathologization and criminalization of the user. Unfortunately, as the poet T. S. Eliot once said, "Between the idea and the reality. Between the motion and the act. Falls the shadow" (from the poem "The Hollow Men"). So, the best intentions have not always been translated into concrete actions.

The PMAQ data made explicit the many problems the country is facing. There are many weak links in the care process: lack of funding, poor administration, insufficient service offer, increase in private sectors' competition for public resources (originally destined for the public sector), lack of commitment of managers and health professionals to the principles of SUS, uneven professional training for SUS professionals, cultural opposition to integration, power conflicts within municipalities, and the predominance of an instrumental-technical mindset to the detriment of a more humane, holistic approach.

Furthermore, problems are not restricted to low coverage in many areas, but especially result from lack of integration of the different facilities and teams working in the same municipality, and of those located in the same health region. To make matters worse, beyond the low coverage and lack of integration between services, there is a clear communication breakdown between what is offered and the demands of the population, particularly for those who do not live in urban centers but in the outskirts of urban areas, in middle-sized and small cities, and in the countryside. This means that, despite the importance of regionalization for optimal functioning of the health care network, difficulties in terms of access and speedy referral, the segmentation of social services, and the fragmentation of care remain major challenges to be properly addressed.

A health system that intends to provide comprehensive management and care must consider the characteristics of living spaces and community dynamics, look at bridges and boundaries, and dive into the structure of the territory and everyday life. Many of the problems made evident by the survey are associated with the lack of knowledge or proper training of people working in the communities and territories. Culturally sensitive programs should be sensitive and flexible in the face of diversity and have the capacity to acknowledge the inadequacy and limits that their practices and conceptual frameworks might have in the face of suffering people with diverse cultural and linguistic codes. This means being able to recognize the different needs of populations in the context of their ethnic and cultural characteristics, as well as their different conceptions about the health–illness process and its relationship with their everyday life and work in their setting. In terms of alcohol and other substances, the territorial dynamics cannot be overlooked.

7.2 Territory and Substance Use

Different fields of knowledge deal with the concepts of territory, thus giving it a wide range of meanings. Like all polysemic terms, it has a variety of interpretations, but consensual definitions have yet to be reached. In the last few years, the concept of territory and its incorporation into the theoretical arsenal and the formulation and monitoring of public policies has gained relevance in the field of public health. The concept of territory represents both a conceptual shift and an operative tool, fostering a better understanding of the health–illness–care process and helping to match policy, planning, and actual interventions with people's lives.

In this scenario, there has been a considerable effort to go beyond reductive views that associate territory exclusively with one of its several dimensions, that is, as a given physical space or one ascribed area (for instance, as a reference for health planning). According to Haesbaert (2004), there are at least three other dimensions when dealing with this concept: politics, culture, and economy. There are many possible theoretical and practical developments and applications of the concept of territory, including materialistic and judicial perspectives, as well as relational and integrative perspectives. In this work, we focus on one perspective, known as the "political ontology of territory" (Escobar 2014), which functions as a counterpoint to perspectives that focus on dualistic worldviews such as human/nonhuman, individual/society, nature/culture, mind/body, secular/holy, and reason/emotion.

Dualistic ontologies, curiously, emerged at the dawn of modernity in a systematic way from René Descartes (1596–1650) and have persisted for many centuries despite consistent criticism of both philosophical and empirical nature. The latter is present for instance in works by Damasio (2003, 2005). Dualism and instrumental rationality do not adequately consider the many ways of living, the existence of different worlds, spatial heterogeneity and its social and symbolic dimensions, or the broad and complex determination of health, illness, suffering, and care.

Territory, therefore, should be viewed as De Certeau defines it, "as a place of practice" (De Certeau 1998). This refers to a dynamic spatiality, constantly updated and activated, which composes and decomposes itself uninterruptedly from its everyday uses and symbolic agencies, narratives and power discourses, cultural practices, and fragments of life stories.

With a political ontology of territory in mind, we need to consider the singularities of the ways of life, affective relations, sociabilities, and bonds between subjects and institutions, which reverberate on the presentation and processes of illness and suffering, as well as in the possibilities of support and care. In this way, it is necessary to understand that the way in which the health–illness–care process becomes a material event in a given territory is the result of an array of factors that occur at several different levels of determination, varying from the most basic interpersonal relations to macrosocial aspects. For Koga,

> To deal with the territorial dimensions brings new elements to the ethical and citizenship debates on public policy and on fighting social exclusion. It asks for the cultural dimension of populations, its local particularities, the places where they live, their yearnings and not only their needs. (Koga 2003, p. 28).

Public health is limited by its incapacity to implement redistributive policies effectively, because it cannot properly handle the diversity and the prevailing inequalities in the territories, restricting itself to specific and predetermined targeted audiences (Koga 2003). In addition, the hypothetical optimal allocation of resources and the "impersonalization" of decision making, for example, in the context of a hypothetical "bureaucratic rationality," as originally formulated by Max Weber (1864–1920), needs to overcome certain constraints. Budget constraints, almost invariably operate in the opposite direction of equity (as there are no powers that can exist without some degree of concentration and a directionality, be it macro, micro or both). Structural vetoes are imposed because of political or administrative instances (on the veto structure under the optics of "policy analysis," we recommend the classic work by Tsebelis (2002)). Hence, the challenge is to make a situational analysis of the social and health needs of a population together with their life conditions, be it in the context of large urban centers or the countryside.

Two publications on the geography of health and health care (Remoaldo and Nogueira 2012; Santana 2014) take territory as a fundamental concept, highlighting the health inequalities, spatial patterns of different health conditions, as well as access and the ways of utilizing health services as elements directly associated with the space characteristics in a broad sense. The authors show that the health profiles of populations depend, to a large extent, on the territory in which they live. This means that health is influenced by the attributes of the context in its physical, social, economic, cultural, and historical dimensions (such as its structure and organization, [lack of] social cohesion, safety/risk, etc.). They conclude by drawing attention to the fact that "health results not only depend on who you are, but where you live" (Remoaldo and Nogueira 2012, p. 21). In this way, every place is a synthesis of multiple interconnected factors that determine its potential to create and perpetuate social inequalities in health or, on the other hand, to be a space where health can thrive in its broadest definitions and consequences.

Santana (2014) highlights an important aspect of the relationship between context and mental health, which concerns the fact that the characteristics of each setting may facilitate or inhibit behaviors, practices, lifestyles, and health and welfare improvements (walking in public spaces, physical exercise, healthy diet, etc.). The author highlights the strong associations between impoverished areas with strong deprivation (in the sense of many interacting hardships, not only economic problems) and mental health. The populations that live in areas deeply affected by poverty and in precarious socio-environmental conditions usually have more difficulties in recognizing the multicausal determination of the health–illness process (given the undeniable strength and dominant character of proximal determinants), are more vulnerable to different risk factors, have less access to health services (especially mental health services), and are prone to be stigmatized, establishing a vicious circle that is very hard to break.

When talking about substance use, there is a long-established tendency to simplify the many dimensions of the phenomena, making the subjects that consume them scapegoats, who are usually labeled as criminals and/or people who are prey to "moral weakness." The latter was the prevalent conception at the end of the nineteenth century and beginning of the twentieth century, under the influence of the temperance movement (the book by Gusfield (1986) gives an analysis of such a dynamic), which resulted in the 18th Amendment to the American Constitution, instituting prohibition and criminalizing the production, distribution, and sale of alcoholic beverages from 1920 to 1933.

However, it is not possible to hide the power and social control strategies that operate under the legitimacy of the hegemonic world policy of drug prohibition. Obviously, this overarching policy does not affect all populations and territories in the same, indiscriminate way, but it is particularly harsh to those who are vulnerable or socially excluded, the outsiders of "civilized" society (i.e., the poor, the immigrants, and different ethnic minorities). The latter can include black people living in the context of multiracial (but still racist) Western societies, ethnic/religious minorities such as Catholics living in countries that follow the Sharia (a Koran-based legislation that criminalizes and punishes alcohol use), and Islamic migrants in countries with a Christian/non-religious majority (Escohotado 1998; Passos and Souza 2011; Alarcon 2012; Luczak et al. 2014).

7.3 Gentrification and Drug Use in Urban Spaces

Big cities have, over the centuries, been places where immigrants tend to settle (Rérat et al. 2010). As a reaction to this process, policy and programs of urban renovation have been instituted as ways to organize spaces, but have resulted in socio-spatial segregation processes. This section highlights the phenomenon of gentrification, a component of this process that has the potential to, among other effects, intensify stigmatization processes directed toward substance users, especially in relation to consumption in public, open spaces by some populations in urban environments.

The definition of "gentrification" remains an object of debate, expressing its polysemic character. There is a relative consensus that it expresses a phenomenon that has occurred in urban spaces in several regions of the planet. Ruth Glass (1912–1990) came up with the term in the 1960s to describe the influx of the new middle classes from the suburbs to central areas in London, UK, after old central buildings, long abandoned, were restored. This influx altered the social composition of the city center, directly or indirectly displacing the working class and the poorest populations that had lived there previously.

Here, we debate the sociospatial segregation that results from this reorganization of urban spaces. Among its consequences is heightening of the stigma related to drug users, despite the existence of an underlying sociability that is often neglected by social and psychological studies.

The emergence of a "new working class," which moves to city regions that have been subject to re-ordination as promoted by urban renovation processes, follows the consolidation of industrial capitalism on the way to post-industrialization. Families comprising this segment of the population are characterized by the presence of women in managerial positions in large corporations, couples with few or no children, employment in the "avant-garde services" sector (e.g. advanced computation, telecommunications), and a high level of education (Shaw 2008; Rérat et al. 2010).

Evictions are often treated in the literature as displacement, an euphemism for the expulsion of poor people from central areas because of commercial interests (real estate corporations, new business) and/or the new middle-class dynamics (Slater 2006; Shaw 2008; Desmond 2017). At the same time that the working class is expelled from these regions, the expansion of consumer and spending capacity makes city centers a magnet for temporary jobs (e.g., watching over cars), sale of low value products (e.g., gums and candies), and drug dealing, once the strong potential of the purchasing power of the middle class is taken into account.

The media often treats the presence of certain populations as undesirable in urban centers, fostering sociospatial stigmatization processes. Davidson and Lees (2005) add that displacement may also have a phenomenological meaning: the loss of a space, of a place or safe haven (neighborhood, community, home, etc.). Reinforcement of the sense of belonging and fostering community development are the keys against the actual and symbolic force of coercive measures (UNODC 2013).

Rérat et al. (2010) argue that emphasis on economic or cultural factors to explain the phenomenon of gentrification also comes from the context in which such explanations emerge. The emblematic work by Smith (1984, 1996) emphasizes economic aspects (based on the Neomarxist matrix) after the intense polarization and emergence of harsh conflicts during the New York gentrification process.

In continental Europe, the renewal and revalorization of historical patrimony have been carried out in sync with attempts to boost tourism and cultural consumption (Gaspar 2010). The growing political autonomy of cities in the context of the global process of economic neoliberalism, which since the 1990s has acted to deregulate markets and shrink the role of the State, has intensified competition between European cities to attract tourists as a key source of revenue and prestige.

Smith (2002, 2006) tells how it is possible to note that gentrified areas go through a real estate price surge, with the subsequent eviction of poorer strata and reduction in cultural and ethnic diversity in the population of the central areas (with an increase in the affluent white middle-class population), and an increase in social inequities and social polarization.

A dimension of social polarization that has been highlighted by several studies is the so-called NIMBY or "not in my backyard" syndrome, a social reaction of urban groups installed in central regions or other highly valued areas when faced with plans to build or develop services and other facilities for the "undesired," such as health services, social services, places offering jobs that might attract the circulation of people seen as dangerous (i.e., those associated by zero-tolerance policies with criminality and violence).

The extreme difficulty of implementing needle and syringe programs in the places where such services are most in need are classic examples of the unfortunate consequences of the NIMBY syndrome and related reactions inspired by racism and marginalization in the USA (Davidson and Howe 2014).

As discussed by Shaw (2008), the key question is not more or less State intervention – there has always been State intervention in urban policy, for good and for bad – but whose interests are heard.

Wacquant (2008) suggests that it is necessary to characterize more precisely the working class that, in the twenty-first century, has been removed, excluded, or evicted from urban centers. There are important morphological changes that must be better understood, taking into account the process of class decomposition, with the consequent de-proletarianization, progressive work informality, and precarization. The author proposes that study of the social structure and everyday life of workers could supply new and important insights, suggesting that people should analyze the structural question of "mass unemployment and its potential impact for the new bureaucratic problematization of 'exclusion' and 'integration'" (Wacquant 2008, p. 54), and look at the desocialization of salaried work as the socioeconomic basis for urban degradation.

The debate about gentrification in Latin America is complex and the very use of the concept has been challenged as a proper tool for explaining the urban renewal processes taking place in the region. To understand the drug trade in these regions asks for an in-depth analysis of the historical dynamics of European colonization in

Latin America. The colonizers imposed an urban pattern and a political and administrative structure in which colonizing powers, their representatives, and institutions embodied the civilizational ideal, whereas the colonized represented the "wild life" to be decimated or subjugated to justify the seizure of assets and the elimination of native peoples (Ianni 1988). African slavery added an extra level/focus of discrimination and conflict that has thrived up to the present, notwithstanding the myth of racial democracy (Domingues 2005; Vieira Pinto 2008). The urban peripheries, especially relevant in the large Latin American urban areas, have channeled the persistent marginalization of impoverished urban populations and their eviction toward poverty enclaves (such as favelas) inside the cities, or toward the outskirts of major urban areas (Maricato 2000).

This marginalized population is either evicted or "contained," as exemplified in inner city São Paulo ("Crackland") and extensively broadcast by different media to international audiences (Lutteroth 2015; Bansal 2014; BBC News 2017). With the inauguration of a new municipal administration in early 2017, new challenges emerged, as described next.

On Sunday 21 May 2017, at dawn (5 h 45 min), the first images of the disastrous removal of people who lived in the Luz central region, also known as "Crackland," were transmitted by the press. The operation was jointly planned by the São Paulo administration, under the direct guidance of the new mayor João Dória and the state of São Paulo's governor, Geraldo Alckmin. At dawn, military troops marched into the region, pushing residents away by throwing tear gas bombs from helicopters flying in circles over this area, with the purpose of breaking by force the so-called "flux": the area frequented by ~600 people in the central region of São Paulo, where purchase of illicit drugs and crack use took place in open scenes. People that lived in the region, dispersed by a violent raid, had to find solace in the region's shelters, which did not have enough beds because they had not being warned this operation would be launched.

On the very same day that the forced removal took place, and continuing on Monday, local properties (households, small businesses) in the region were vacated (also by force) and "sealed," which meant that brick walls were erected in front of their doors and windows so that the people who lived there could no longer get inside. On Tuesday, buildings characterized as of "public interest" were demolished. During the demolition, some of the debris hit a nearby building, injuring three people.

A short time after the operation, the Public Defender's Office denounced the lack of dialogue with the population (meaning both the users and nearby residents) throughout the process, generating insecurity about what would follow. On Wednesday (24 May 2017) the Public Defender obtained a legal mandate that forbade removals to continue. The mayor and governor planned a press conference after cancellation of the operation, but the press conference did not take place. Later, neither managers hid the immediate motive of the operation: they claimed that crack addiction was very complex and few users accepted treatment, but that the key point was that the region known as Crackland no longer existed. However, one week after the operation, 23 new spots of crack consumption were identified in the region as surrogates of the original that clustered around Santa Isabel Square.

In parallel with forced removals, the end of the program "De Braços Abertos" (DBA) [Open Arms] was announced. The DBA was inspired by the initiatives of the first housing programs. Sam Tsemberis, attributed with the original formulation of the "Housing First" proposal, said that in the USA, since the Reagan administration, there are homeless people whose situation has become chronic in ways never seen before. Such initiatives have been proven successful in several countries besides America, such as Australia, Canada, Finland, France, and Japan. The principles on which the DBA is based are as follows: comprehensive care integrated with social welfare initiatives and health promotion, harm reduction, reinforcement of subjects' autonomy, and job offer as well as housing. DBA was managed by a board composed of the civil society, non-governmental organizations (NGOs) that worked with homeless people, and representatives of the people who use alcohol and other substances.

The network of professional psychology boards, composed of the Conselho Federal de Psicologia (CFP) [Federal Psychology Council] and its 23 regional boards, sent out a note repudiating the violent police raid, appealing to people and institutions working with human rights and the legislation regulating Brazilian psychiatric reform.

A key component of the mayor's initiative was involuntary, compulsory psychiatric hospitalization or referral to religious-based "therapeutic communities." Several political analysts have highlighted the fact that the biggest beneficiary of police operations targeting crack users and local residents is the real estate sector, which intends to gentrify the region under the aegis of the municipal administration (Gonçalves 2011).

7.4 Alcohol and Substances Policy: Dissonances in the Context of Rural Communities

Studies and publications on rural populations, specifically on substance use, are still scarce in Brazil, unlike other countries, where the issue is already an object of peer-reviewed journals dedicated to this theme (e.g., *The Journal of Rural Health*; available at http://onlinelibrary.wiley.com/journal/10.1111/(ISSN)1748-0361). At first, it seems that resources such as peer-reviewed journals and regular research are a privilege of high-income countries such as the USA and Australia. However, this is a totally wrong point of view because the scientific production and practical initiatives of low-income countries facing serious economic problems (such as Cuba) have been particularly strong, as documented by the World Health Organization (2008).

Most studies analyzing the health of these populations focus on the morbidities associated with multiple and intermittent application of pesticides, among which are psychiatric conditions and suicide attempts, as well as effects secondary to technological changes in the farming processes and accidents associated with innovative working processes. Obviously, such questions are relevant, not only from the public health point of view, but also from the perspective of the failure of public power in its duty to regulate and carry out monitoring and surveillance on a continuous basis. As an example, major problems are documented in the extensive dossier recently issued by the Associação Brasileira de Saúde Coletiva (ABRASCO) [Brazilian Collective Health Association] (ABRASCO 2015).

In addition, traditional approaches are usually reinforced by oversimplistic conceptions about rural space, anchored in the imaginary notion that the urban and the rural are completely distinctive realities in which the first represents the past, the residual, whereas the latter is the advanced and modern opposite pole. Nothing could be more distant from reality in a country where agribusiness represents the largest share of the gross domestic product (GDP), with substantial mechanization of many crops (e.g., soybean) and the processing in situ of many commodities (see different analyses available in the *Revista USP* dossier on rural issues; Revista USP 2005).

Scholars such as Wanderley discuss the "emergence of a new rural" (Wanderley 2000, p. 90) marked by the development of local industrial processing plants; the diversity of social actors that establish new relations with the soil, machines, processes and semi-industrial commodities; and the emergence of new political actors in the field.

In this scenario, city and the countryside are increasingly interconnected and affected by challenges and dilemmas that may jeopardize the traditional structure and processes of both settings and determine major alterations in both, irrespective of their undeniable specificities. In this way, it is important to analyze differences and connections, gaps and bottlenecks, and continuities and discontinuities between the urban and the rural from the perspective of the evolving historical and social dynamics.

Furthermore, when considering the diversity of social groups that compose the rural population of Brazil, comprising small and medium-sized farms, big land owners, and small family-owned businesses, but also extractivists (forest people, agro-extractivists, *ribeirinhos* [river margins settlers], artisanal fishermen and crab collectors), cashew collectors, *babaçu* extractivists, açaí planters, small tenants, informal partners, renters, *quilombolas* [descendants of the historical antislavery black resistance], members of indigenous tribes, *serranos* [hill people], *cablocos* [multiracial populations], as well people from the country's southern border of mixed (Portuguese/Spanish) descent (Godoi et al. 2009).

It is necessary to acknowledge the different needs, strengths, and vulnerabilities, as well as diverse life conditions and social organization levels of those people. Such diversity determines particular living styles and occupations, different types of sociability and social identities, and different ways to understand health and illness, which shape the physical territories as well as the existential trajectories of these populations. In this way, the rural environment cannot be understood as a mere physical space where the production and lives of inhabitants take place, but the outcome of complex living styles, social interactions, and cultural expressions (Otero 2013).

Regardless of that, it is known that the vulnerability secondary to poverty and sparse/absent/hard-to-reach services is much worse in rural spaces (compared with metropolitan areas), keeping in mind the huge disparity between its different segments (varying from small family-owned businesses to megasized agribusiness complexes). Socioeconomic indicators reveal that the rural areas have not yet been freed from major hurdles and gaps such as a considerable level of illiteracy, food insecurity, high infant mortality (compared with the current standards of urban Brazil), difficulty in accessing public services and technical help, precarious work conditions, and more dependency on income transference programs. Dire life conditions persist, sometimes side-by-side with advanced capitalist enterprises (that actually profit from such a vast pool of underemployed people), despite the advances of social policies and interventions implemented by many rural social movements such as MST (the landless movement), the rural union movement, and several NGOs, associations, and cooperatives.

Residents still suffer from exposure to climatic instability in several regions such as the Northeast (probably aggravated by ongoing global warming), due to very dry seasons or catastrophic floods; the lack of natural resources in some areas, such as the hinterlands of some northeastern states; and the non-implementation and/or bad use of agricultural credit and precarious transportation. The pressing need to develop emergency strategies to complement meager family incomes compromises collective organization and political participation, thus aborting opportunities to empower themselves and change the local standards of development, health, and community life. Environmental degradation, exposure to pesticides, poor diet, lack of leisure spaces, low levels of social support, and the very high workload in both rural and domestic contexts among women have been associated with high rates of chronically degenerative illnesses, including the presence of psychiatric morbidities and harmful/dependent alcohol/drug use among men and women (sometimes also affecting minors). It is worth noticing here that no other geographic context in Brazil has such a dangerous combination of chronic-degenerative illnesses and classic infectious illnesses, both endemic and epidemic (e.g., malaria, schistosomiasis, and, more recently, emerging and re-emerging illnesses such as chikungunya and yellow fever).

From the perspective of public policies, there is a clear priority for urban spaces in detriment of rural areas, which is not only unfair, but economically and socially disastrous.

Concerning the National Mental Health Policy, besides the dire picture we have discussed here, particularly for the smaller municipalities with characteristically rural features, there is no established directive of care and attention for rural populations, despite the fact that they constitute a collective with specific needs and demands, deeply embedded into concrete life and working conditions.

Even in the context of the most recent public policy, which focused on integral health to be delivered to rural and forest populations (Brazilian Ministry of Health 2011b), there are no references to mental health associated with the territorial, social, and sociocultural particularities that may characterize the specific ways of life of these populations and, consequently, their specific health needs and particular ways of understanding health, illness, and care. Such references are also needed to guide the planning and provision of care, such as the offer of management and care guided by a psychosocial framework. For Bosi and Guerriero, to recognize these aspects "demands dedicated professionals to promote serious reflection and collective efforts toward a deeper understanding of the complexity of the setting they have been working with" (Bosi and Guerriero 2016, p. 139).

In the context of (potential) networks of psychosocial care (RAPS), the health care for rural and forest populations facing mental suffering and harms and risks associated with the use of crack, alcohol and other substances remains sparse and poorly integrated (most of the so-called networks should not be denominated as such).

Rural populations face serious problems of access when it comes to health equipment, do not benefit from proper coverage by the Programa de Agentes Comunitários de Saúde (PACS) [Community Health Agents Program] and the Estratégia de Saúde da Família (ESF) [Strategy for Family Health]. This also applies to the teams located in the Núcleos de Apoio à Saúde da Família (NASF) [Family Support Hubs], which have been providing a very modest coverage to rural areas. In addition to the lack of knowledge of territorial particularities, there is a shortage of professionals and the absence of true multidisciplinary teams (Guimarães et al. 2014; Santana 2014). These problems are combined with precarious organization and management of services, long waiting lines, restricted treatment hours, and stigmatizing and moralistic attitudes toward mentally ill users, particularly those individuals with special needs associated with the harmful/dependent use of alcohol and other substances.

To give an example of our reasoning, we selected data on primary care service access by populations in rural settlements and *quilombola* communities in Brazil from PMAQ's statements and norms (Macedo et al. 2017). By rural settlements, we understand a group of agricultural hubs that, according to government policies based on programs and prospects of agrarian reform, aim to ensure decent housing conditions and boost family production, as well as seek new social patterns in the development of agricultural processes and community life (Bergamasco and Norder 1996).

According to the Instituto Nacional de Colonização e Reforma Agrária (INCRA) [National Institute for Colonization and Agrarian Reform], there are at least 9357 settlement projects all over the national territory, benefiting about 974,505 families. As for the *quilombola* communities, ethnic groups formed by rural black populations (sometimes urban remnants, which goes beyond the scope of this text), whose social identity is made from their relations with the soil, kinship, their centuries-long territories, ancestrality, and their own cultural practices (Schmitt et al. 2002). About 2474 remaining *quilombola* communities have been recognized by the Brazilian state, and other 1533 communities have launched applications to become certified according to the current legislation.

By comparative analysis of the localities where rural settlements and *quilombola* communities are located versus the municipalities where the 17,482 health teams researched in PMAQ are working, it was possible to observe that 5970 teams (34.14%) deal with a population that lives in settlement areas and 3625 teams (21.10%) work with populations that live in *quilombola* communities. The most relevant (and deeply frustrating) finding of this quick survey was that only 1965 of the teams that participated in the PMAQ evaluation answered questions about health care to rural settlements and/or *quilombolas*. Of these, 73.7% answered that they had not performed actions directed to these communities; a meager 8.7% of the global set of health teams benefited from transportation to deliver assistance to these communities; and only 10.3% reported that they managed at least the more critical cases from such areas (Macedo et al. 2017).

This is a bleak picture, documenting lack of proper health care, despite the approval of a national policy specifically issued to guarantee the health of rural and forest populations, nationally known as "Saúde Integral das Populações do Campo e da Floresta" (PNSIPCF). The structural bottlenecks and the scarcity of resources and manpower have hindered the translation of such policies into concrete initiatives.

Recent research, carried out in rural settlements in two northeastern states of Brazil (Dimenstein et al. 2016) on the patterns of alcohol use in settlements targeted by agrarian reform, has evidenced how much poor life conditions and unequal social and gender relations remain as key factors associated with the problematic use of alcohol in these contexts. We observed marked differences in drinking habits between men and women, to the detriment of disenfranchised women. Education seems to be a protective element, opening new paths to other, renewed life projects. Additional factors pose serious constraints, such as the persistent difficulties in accessing facilities and services or the absence of spaces for leisure/coexistence.

There is still much to be developed in terms of public policies and, especially, their translation into concrete improvements, such as the need for specific guidelines for rural populations regarding mental health and the use of substances. The investment in mental health care in the frame of a territory-based policy, fostering proximity and dialogue, as well as the integration of mental health care into primary care is fundamental for reorientation of professional practices and attitudes. It is crucial that the services of health and social protection fit territorial dynamics, as well as the social, cultural, and labor specificities of the rural context, always keeping in mind the parallel persistence of traditional practices within historical communities, as well as the deep transformations and changes in the rural contexts and their implications for mental health management and care.

References

Alarcon, S. (Org.). (2012). Álcool e outras drogas: diálogos sobre uma mal-estar contemporâneo. Rio de Janeiro: Fiocruz.

ABRASCO. (2015). Dossiê Associação Brasileira de Saúde Coletiva (ABRASCO). *Um alerta sobre os impactos dos* agrotóxicos *na saúde*. Rio de Janeiro and São Paulo: EPSJV and Expressão Popular. Retrieved from http://www.abrasco.org.br/dossieagrotoxicos/wp-content/uploads/2013/10/DossieAbrasco_2015_web.pdf

Bansal, S. (2014, October 29). Controversial São Paulo project offers jobs to crack addicts in Cracolândia. *The Guardian*. Retrieved from https://www.theguardian.com/global-development/2014/oct/29/sao-paulo-brazil-crack-addicts-drugs

BBC News. (2017, May 21). Brazil police raid Sao Paulo 'Crackland' and make arrests. *BBC News*. Retrieved from http://www.bbc.com/news/world-latin-america-39994177

Becker, H. (1997). *Outsiders: Studies in the sociology of deviance*. New York: Free Press.

Bergamasco, S. M. P. P., & Norder, L. A. C. (1996). *O que são assentamentos rurais?* São Paulo: Brasiliense.

Bolonheis-Ramos, R. C. M., & Boarini, M. L. (2015). Therapeutic communities: "New" outlooks and public health proposals. *História, Ciências, Saúde-Manguinhos, 22*(4), 1231–1248. https://doi.org/10.1590/S0104-59702015000400005.

Bosi, M. L. M. S., & Guerriero, I. Z. (2016). Desafios éticometodológicos nas pesquisas em saúde mental com populações vulneráveis. In M. Dimenstein, J. Leite, J. P. Macedo, & C. Dantas (Eds.), *Condições de Vida e Saúde Mental em Contextos Rurais* (pp. 121–140). São Paulo and Brasília: Editora Intermeios and CNPQ.

Brazilian Ministry of Health. (2003). Ministério da Saúde. Secretaria Executiva. Coordenação Nacional de DST/Aids. *A Política do Ministério da Saúde para atenção integral a usuários de álcool e outras drogas*. Brasília: Ministério da Saúde. Retrieved from http://bvsms.saude.gov.br/bvs/publicacoes/politica_atencao_alcool_drogas.pdf

Brazilian Ministry of Health. (2011a). Ministério da Saúde. *Portaria N° 3.088, de 23 de dezembro de* 2011. Rede de Atenção Psicossocial para pessoas com sofrimento ou transtorno mental e com necessidades decorrentes do uso de crack, álcool e outras drogas, no âmbito do Sistema Único de Saúde (SUS). Brasília: Ministério de Saúde.

Brazilian Ministry of Health. (2011b). Ministério da Saúde. *Política nacional de saúde integral às populações do campo e da floresta*. Brasília: SEGP

Chiaverni, D. H. (Ed.). (2011). *Guia prático de matriciamento em saúde mental*. Brasília: Ministério da Saúde.

Damasio, A. (2003). *Looking for Spinoza: Joy, sorrow, and the feeling brain*. Orlando, FL: Harvest Books.

Damasio, A. (2005). *Descartes' error: Emotion, reason, and the human brain*. London: Penguin Books.

Davidson, M., & Lees, L. (2005). New-build gentrification and London's riverside renaissance. *Environment and Planning, 37*(7), 1165–1190.

Davidson, P. J., & Howe, M. (2014). Beyond NIMBYism: Understanding community antipathy toward needle distribution services. *The International Journal on Drug Policy, 25*(3), 624–632.

De Certeau, M. (1998). *A invenção do cotidiano: as artes de fazer*. Petrópolis: Vozes.

Desmond, M. (2017). *Evicted: Poverty and profit in the American city*. New York: Broadway Books.

Dimenstein, M., Leite, J. F., Macedo, J. P., & Dantas, C. (Eds.). (2016). *Condições de vida e saúde mental em contextos rurais*. São Paulo and Brasília: Intermeios and CNPQ.

Domingues, P. (2005). O mito da democracia racial e a mestiçagem no Brasil (1889-1930). *Diálogos Latinoamericanos, 10*, 116–131.

Duarte, L. F. (1986). *Da vida nervosa (nas classes trabalhadoras urbanas)*. Rio de Janeiro: Jorge Zahar Editor/CNPQ.

Escobar, A. (2014). *Sentipensar con la tierra: nuevas lecturas sobre desarrollo, territorio y diferencia*. Medellín: Unaula.

Escohotado, A. (1998). *Historia de las drogas*. Barcelona: Alianza.

Friedman, P., Des Jarlais, D. C., Peyser, N. P., Nichols, S. E., Drew, E., & Newman, R. G. (1994). Retention of patients who entered methadone maintenance via an interim methadone clinic. *Journal of Psychoactive Drugs, 26*(2), 217–221.

Gaspar, S. S. (2010). Gentrification: processo global, especificidades locais? *Ponto Urbe, 6*, 1–16. Retrieved from http://pontourbe.revues.org/1575.

Godoi, E. P., Menezes, M. A., & Marin, R. A. (Eds.). (2009). *Diversidade do campesinato: Expressões e categorias. Vol. 2: Estratégias de reprodução social*. São Paulo: Editora UNESP.

Goffman, E. (1961). *Asylums: Essays on the social situation of mental patients and other inmates*. New York: Anchor Books/Doubleday.

Gonçalves, A. M. (2002). Cuidados diante do abuso e da dependência de drogas: desafio da prática do Programa Saúde da Família (Doctoral dissertation, Universidade de São Paulo, Ribeirão Preto).

Gonçalves, G. A. (2011). Reclassification of the downtown area of São Paulo. *Estudos Avançados, 25*(71), 109–118.

Guimarães, R. B., Pickenhayn, J. A., & Lima, S. C. (2014). *Geografia e saúde sem fronteiras*. Uberlândia: Editora Assis.

Gusfield, J. R. (1986). *Symbolic crusade: Status politics and the American temperance movement*. Urbana and Chicago: University of Illinois Press.

Haesbaert, R. (2004). *O mito da desterritorialização*. Rio de Janeiro: Bertrand Brasil.

História, Ciências, Saúde – Manguinhos. (2013). Falta de médicos é o maior problema do SUS? *História, Ciências, Saúde – Manguinhos* July 2013. Retrieved from http://www.revistahcsm.coc.fiocruz.br/falta-de-medicos-e-o-maior-problema-do-sus

Ianni, O. (1988). A questão nacional na América Latina. *Estudos Avançados, 2*(1), 5–40. https://doi.org/10.1590/S0103-40141988000100003.

Koga, D. (2003). *Medidas de cidades: entre territórios de vida e territórios vividos*. São Paulo: Cortez.

Luczak, S. E., Prescott, C. A., Dalais, C., Raine, A., Venables, P. H., & Mednick, S. A. (2014). Religious factors associated with alcohol involvement: Results from the Mauritian Joint Child Health Project. *Drug and Alcohol Dependence, 135*, 37–44.

Lutteroth, V. J. (2015, April 10). Aus dem Dunkeln geholt [Out of the dark]. *Die Spiegel*. Retrieved from http://www.spiegel.de/panorama/gesellschaft/rio-de-janeiro-crack-suechtige-in-ein-drucksvoller-fotoserie-a-1027602.html

Macedo, J. P., Abreu, M. M., & Dimenstein, M. (2017). *Relatório Parcial de Pesquisa. Regionalização da Assistência em Álcool e Drogas no Brasil*. Parnaíba: UFPI.

Maricato, E. (2000). Urbanismo na periferia do mundo globalizado: metrópoles brasileiras. *São Paulo em Perspectiva, 14*(4), 21–33. https://doi.org/10.1590/S0102-88392000000400004.

Otero, M. (2013). Prefácio IICA. In C. Miranda & H. Silva (Eds.), *Concepções da ruralidade contemporânea: as singularidades brasileiras. Vol. 21: Série Desenvolvimento Rural Sustentável* (pp. 13–14). Brasília: Instituto Interamericano de Cooperação para a Agricultura. Retrieved from http://repiica.iica.int/DOCS/B3226P/B3226P.PDF.

Passos, E. H., & Souza, T. P. (2011). Redução de danos e saúde pública: construções alternativas à política global de "guerra às drogas". *Psicologia & Sociedade, 23*(1), 154–162. https://doi.org/10.1590/S0102-71822011000100017.

Remoaldo, P., & Nogueira, H. (2012). Variações e desigualdades socioterritoriais em saúde. Capítulo 1. In: *Desigualdades socioterritoriais e comportamentos em saúde*. Lisboa: Edições Colibri.

Rérat, P., Söderström, O., & Piguet, E. (2010). New forms of gentrification: Issues and debates. *Population, Space and Place, 16*, 335–343. https://doi.org/10.1002/psp.585.

Revista USP. (2005). Dossiê Brasil Rural, 64, 6–173. Retrieved from http://www.revistas.usp.br/revusp/issue/view/1065?

Rosenstock, K. I. V., & Neves, M. J. (2010). Papel do enfermeiro da atenção básica de saúde na abordagem ao dependente de drogas em João Pessoa, PB, Brasil. *Revista Brasileira de Enfermagem, 63*(4), 581–586. https://doi.org/10.1590/S0034-71672010000400013.

Santana, P. (2014). *Introdução à geografia da saúde: território, saúde e bem-estar*. Coimbra: Coimbra University Press.

Saraceno, B., van Ommeren, M., Batniji, R., Cohen, A., Gureje, O., Mahoney, J., Sridhar, D., & Underhill, C. (2007). Barriers to improvement of mental health services in low-income and middle-income countries. *Lancet, 370*(9593), 1164–1174.

Schmitt, A., Turatti, M. C. M., & Carvalho, M. C. P. (2002). A atualização do conceito de quilombo: identidade e território nas definições teóricas. *Ambiente & Sociedade, 10*, 129–136. https://doi.org/10.1590/S1414-753X2002000100008.

Shaw, K. (2008). Gentrification: What it is, why it is, and what can be done about it. *Geography Compass, 2*, 1697–1728. https://doi.org/10.1111/j.1749-8198.2008.00156.x.

Silveira, M. R. (2009). *A saúde mental na atenção básica: um diálogo necessário*. Doctoral thesis, Universidade Federal de Minas Gerais, Belo Horizonte.

Slater, T. (2006). The eviction of critical perspectives from gentrification research. *International Journal of Urban and Regional Research, 30*, 737–757. https://doi.org/10.1111/j.1468-2427.2006.00689.x.

Smith, N. (1984). *Uneven development: Nature, capital and the production of space*. Oxford: Blackwell.

Smith, N. (1996). *The new urban frontier: Gentrification and the revanchist city*. London and New York: Routledge.

Smith, N. (2002). New globalism, new urbanism: Gentrification as global urban strategy. *Antipode, 3*, 427–450.

Smith, N. (2006). A gentrificação generalizada: de uma anomalia local à "regeneração" urbana como estratégia urbana global. In C. Bidou-Zachariansen, D. Hiernaux-Nicolas, & H. Rivière d'Arc (Eds.), *De volta à cidade: dos processos de gentrificação às políticas de "revitalização" dos centros urbanos*. São Paulo: Annablume.

Starfield, B. (2002). Atenção Primária: equilíbrio entre necessidades de saúde, serviços e tecnologia. Brasília: UNESCO, Ministério da Saúde.

Tavares, A. L. B., Souza, A. R., & Pontes, R. J. S. (2013). Estudo da demanda de saúde mental em Centro de Saúde da Família em Caucaia, Ceará, Brasil. *Revista Brasileira de Medicina de Família e Comunidade, 8*(26), 35–42. https://doi.org/10.5712/rbmfc8(26)492.

Tsebelis, G. (2002). *Veto players: How political institutions work*. Princeton, NJ: Princeton University Press.

UNODC. (2013). *Da_coercao_a_coesao_portugues [From coercion to cohesion. Treating drug dependence through health care, not punishment]*. Vienna: United Nations Office on Drugs and Crime. Retrieved from https://www.unodc.org/documents/lpobrazil/noticias/2013/09/Da_coercao_a_coesao_portugues.pdf.

Vieira Pinto, A. (2008). *A sociologia dos países subdesenvolvidos*. Rio de Janeiro: Contraponto.

Wacquant, L. (2008). *Punishing the poor: The neoliberal government of social insecurity*. Durham, NC and London: Duke University Press.

Wanderley, M. N. B. (2000). A emergência de uma nova ruralidade nas sociedades modernas avançadas – o "rural" como espaço singular e ator coletivo. *Estudos Sociedade e Agricultura, 15*, 87–145.

World Health Organization. (2008). *La revolución de la atención primaria en Cuba cumple 30 años*. Geneva: WHO. Retrieved from http://www.who.int/bulletin/volumes/86/5/08-030508/es/.

Yancovitz, S. R., Des Jarlais, D. C., Peyser, N. P., Drew, E., Friedmann, P., Trigg, H. L., & Robinson, J. W. (1991). A randomized trial of an interim methadone maintenance clinic. *American Journal of Public Health, 81*(9), 1185–1191.

Index

T. M. Ronzani (ed.), *Drugs and Social Context*,
https://doi.org/10.1007/978-3-319-72446-1

Printed by Printforce, the Netherlands